I0115701

FAT CONFESSIONALS

This book is the result of almost 28 years of an emotional- eating and couch-sitting lifestyle. It wasn't an afterthought and it didn't happen overnight. As humiliating as these confessionals are, my hope is that by putting them to paper, someone else out there who might be trapped in that lifestyle can find their way out of it like I did. Many thanks to the followers of my little blog that started on Facebook for giving me the confidence to share my confessions publicly and for reminding me daily that I am not the only emotional eater in the world and that my truths can help many others.

The confessions you are about to read are completely true are not listed in any particular order… these confessions would not be possible without the following: mac 'n' cheese, cake and cake frosting of all kinds, french fries, pizza, the couch, my excuses, the remote control, chocolate and peanut butter can't forget the peanut butter!

Copyright © 2014 by Caitlin Flora

*   *   *

Fat Confessional #1:

(Frosting)

One of my earliest memories growing up was of the most delicious vanilla frosted cupcakes my mom baked. As soon as they were frosted and placed in the fridge, I would quietly sneak downstairs, open the fridge door and gaze at the cupcakes as if they were the only food left on Earth. Then I would blissfully and slowly lick the icing off each and every one of them, wrap them and replace them on the shelf again.   I still can hear my mom to this day asking me if I ate the icing and me really thinking I could get away with it!! Now? Yes, I still love vanilla icing and anything vanilla in general, but I just stick with vanilla protein powder if I'm craving something sweet or a small glass of vanilla almond milk! Works for me!

*   *   *

Fat Confessional #2

(Fast food addict)

I used to hit the "drive thru" at my local fast food joint and order 3 large, very large hamburger or chicken meals complete with french fries... with sprite, diet coke and coke. I would happily drive off to park somewhere secluded and ditch the sprite and coke, keeping the diet coke and eating all the meals by myself-yes! All by myself!! Why get 3 drinks, you ask? Well, that way I could fool the employees at the restaurant into thinking those meals weren't all for me!! As if they cared about the details of my burger order! As if I thought I'd be put into a burger line-up or something...or get arrested for consuming too many bad foods. As if they didn't already realize I was enormous for a reason and hear my laughter as I asked for extra napkins and ketchup for the "kids" because that food wasn't all for me!! Fast forward to today: I haven't been in any fast food lines for at least a year and counting and you know what? I don't miss it at all. I've found that the less I have of something the less I crave it in the first place. Be strong and don't give in to fast food temptations.

Fat Confessional #3

(Dirty jeans dreams)

At 300 lbs, I hated how tight my freshly washed
and dried jeans were. The chafing and pinching of
the denim was a daily thing. To deal with that, I
would wear my jeans as long as I could. No
washing and drying them for me! Gross, right!!?
My jeans would relax and so would I! But now,
because my much skinnier jeans are falling off me,
I'll throw them in the dryer to make them tighter
again! The snug feeling is something I like to feel
now! How funny is that! The days of struggling
whilst lying down on my pink canopy bed trying to
zipper my pants are over!!

* * *

Fat confessional #4:

(Silly little bad habits)

When you live as large as I did you try everything
but healthy eating and exercise first. You name it I
tried it. Every diet pill over the counter promised
to get me thin without any side effects and only
good results would happen to me. NOT!!!! I never

got the results I wanted and instead ended up with anxiety and a racing heart. Do not mess with any diet pills they may help at first but they will never keep you satisfied. Every diet out there I have tried and I consider myself to be quite the weight loss junkie. Always looking for bigger and better things and better results. Never getting the results I wanted I decided that I would just embrace my fluffery and those E cup boobs of mine that smack me in the face when running...after all I didn't deserve success only failure. My thought process is only just now getting healthy. I tried meal replacement shakes, and loved the vanilla-flavored ones so much that I would drink them often. But I didn't use diet shakes as meal replacements. Instead, I'd have one AFTER -consuming a large regular meal-as a dessert replacement-not as a meal replacement! Kind of defeats the purpose, does it not? Two dinners rolled into one...my dream!!

*   *   *

Fat confessional #5:

(Denial train)

Whenever I was asked about my weight and how I got to weighing over 300 pounds in the first place,

I would always say, " I don't know because I don't eat that much!" I said it so often that I believed it even though no one else did! I guess you could say I was lying to myself as much as I was to everyone else. But that's what it was: a HUGE LIE!! What was I REALLY doing? Well, I would drink a gallon of milk in one day and polish off a large pizza and still want dessert!! That's what I was doing for real! So quit lying to yourself and everyone else!! You know how you got this way and you know what it takes to get fit. So get off the denial train and just do it already!!!

*   *   *

Fat confessional #6:

(Nice rack)

If you have large boobs and hate it stand up...raise your hand and give me a high five because I feel the same way. Those of us with large boobs hate them and those smaller chested ladies sure know how to stick together and wished they had boobs. But how about after spending money sometimes even over $50 on a bra finding the underwire of the bra in the laundry machine. Those stupid bra's are never made the way should be. So here you've spent so much on one item you neglect throwing it away and wear it anyways...so now you're dealing with one boob raised to your chin like a model and the other boob practically sweeping the floor. Well played lingerie stores well played. One boob would have cuts and scrapes directly underneath not to mention permanent marks to show off that you frankly shouldn't have worn the bra without support on both sides. Those darn underwire bras!!!!

Fat Confessional #7:

(No pictures please)

When you live life large many things that are normal for some are not for us. Pictures were always the devil and I always hated having them taken. Now you can't keep me away from selfies but frankly it's because I hated myself so much and made funny jokes about myself or my friends instead. When you poke fun at yourself you don't realize what you're actually doing or saying. You learn to know your surroundings...so that way if you have to find a tree to hide around you do it. You stand behind people in photos so that way they can't see just how big you are. Or you surround yourself with people just as large as you so that way you don't have to be the biggest chick in the group. But pictures aren't the only thing that normal people don't mind. This here is a little TMI but it's hard to shave and clean yourself and even use the bathroom properly without your weight getting in the way. So there ya have it...those are just some of the reasons why I cannot stand to even think of my former fat memories. I'm just so glad my life has changed. You can change your life too ya know..it takes time, patience, strength, hope, determination and a workout buddy doesn't hurt either. Just remember all the horrible things you have to go through when you are over 300 pounds and this should be your motivation to get you started or keep you on the right track. DO NOT FALTER!

Fat confessional #8:
(every fat girl has her tricks)

Ever since I can remember, I've tried never, ever to have my picture taken! I'd hide away from that nasty camera flash, or insist that they (anyone with the camera!) take my pictures from the neck up ONLY because I was humiliated by myself! Really? Yes, I was totally embarrassed and humiliated by my appearance! I would wear all things black and avoid white and bright colors, or anything with horizontal stripes. I used to cry desperately when I couldn't see my own feet in the shower when I looked down!!! Now that I'm a runner, I can give into my cravings! For burgers and desserts? No, for vegetables and healthy whole foods!   And I can finally see my belly button when I look down- without moving a roll to view it!   Never give up, people! Never! I was the least motivated person in the world! But once I changed my way of thinking, my motivation changed too! So bring on the camera folks! And you can do it! You can re-motivate too!!

*   *   *

Fat confessional #9:

(Granny panties)

Yes it's hard to discuss this but I pride myself in my honesty with you all. And yes I'm well aware that those are granny panties but the truth is they are falling off me and that is awesome. Is my body perfect?? Nope. (Photo posted on blog page) I still have stretch marks I still have cellulite I still have loose skin. but I don't care...this body got me to the point that I'm at today.. it's these legs that have taken the steps that have picked the farthest parking spot.. that have walked and ran a million miles.. that took the stairs instead of the elevator. its this body that chose to do it the hard way and never once gave up. I love this body that I have and all the battle wounds left to remind me that I don't ever want to fight that battle again

Fat confessional# 10:

(battle wounds)

My legs feel like a ton of bricks..do I still have cellulite..yes a ton..do I still have loose skin on my thighs..yes a ton..but its slowly getting tighter and tighter..one thing I still can't get used to is my thighs not rubbing together..that's what I think about when temptation arises! I'm odd today so I'm training a friend in another

* * * *

Fat Confessional #11:

(Bent over and can't get back up)

Back when I was over 300 pounds, if I was in a large grocery store or doing any kind of shopping, and if I accidentally dropped something, I'd play "kick the can" and tap it with my foot down the aisle. Or I'd just walk away quickly. Did I just enjoy the fancy footwork? No, I did that because I knew how painful it was to bend over and pick it up!! My legs and back were so stressed with all the weight they had to carry! Sorry to all the hard working employees that had to pick up after me!! And I know it sounds silly but I used to be jealous of women who could cross their legs when they were sitting. Because the truth is that at 300 pounds I could not! One leg wouldn't fit over another no matter how I shifted or positioned myself! It's not a big thing really, but it's those little things that I remember most!

*   *   *

Fat confessional #12:

(track track track)

The saying "you are what you eat"-very true indeed! If you work out hard and challenge yourself and still you see no results, there's only one other thing to do: look at the food on your plate! You'll see then that the real challenge is in the kitchen, not the gym. You'll need a solution like the one I've found that works for me: I suggest you try keeping a Food Journal for 7 days to see where you are going wrong. Keeping a food journal and making small changes each day will finally bring you the results you're looking for! It's a tricky thing dealing with our body. If we eat to little, we won't lose weight and yet if we eat to much, we don't lose either. Just really think about what you're putting into your body before you sit down for a bite.

Fat confessional #13:

(Happy Birthday to me?)

CAKE...ICING…BUTTER CREAM FROSTING…You name it…Cake has my flipping name all over it!!!!! But it's not just ANY cake that'll do, it's the grocery cake with the butter cream frosting that opens the key to my heart like nobody ever could (sorry honey)! For those of you who aren't familiar with butter cream icing on a yellow cake at our local grocery stores…well it's your loss!!!! And for today's "Fat Confessional" I'm revealing my bakery cake strategy, so listen up! This is a good one!! I'll never forget making that phone call to order the birthday cake at the store bakery. It had to include lots of colorful flowers and be the best tasting cake ever!! So I decided to call in and order it, just like that! A yellow cake with butter cream frosting all over it, with pretty pink flowers (extra flowers!). I ordered a 1/4 sheet cake- about 20 servings I was told- and I thought, "That's the perfect size!!" They then asked me if I wanted any filling for the cake, but I said, "No." Better to just go with the yellow cake, no filling needed. After all, not everyone loves fillings in cakes. I let the nice cake lady on the phone know that it was for a birthday and could it please say "Happy Birthday Rachel!" She agreed with my order requirements, and I merrily went out to pick up my treat two days later, so excited to see just how delectable it looked-of course it looked delish! Practically skipping out to my car with the cake, well, skipping isn't easy for an uncoordinated 300 pound girl, but you get the point. I skipped out to my car and drove home. So excited!! Not for a party, but because there was no Rachel!! The cake was for me and me alone!! Rachel was just an imaginary "friend" for my purposes! It wasn't my birthday, but it was my cake-eating party! I will not say that I ate it all in one day, but within a few short days, it was completely consumed. To this day, walking past a store bakery, I still have to practically hold my nose and put my blinders on so I don't give in to the temptation!! After all, Marie Antoinette supposedly said, "Let them Eat Cake!" She did not say, "Hey Cait! Eat all that cake!"

*   *   *

Fat confessional #14:

(Fast food job= food addict gone crazy)

Some of you who are my personal friends may remember that my first job at age 15 was working at a large fast food chain restaurant. I know, I know, the perfect place for a large teenage girl who adores french fries, right?? Right! So I almost always worked weekends, and I would go into work right when the breakfast menu was switching over to the lunch menu for the day. Way back when (wow, over 15 years ago!) the restaurant did not make "fresh food" to order, but instead they would make large quantities of burgers, chicken sandwiches, etc.etc. When the breakfast shift switched over at lunchtime, they would always dump the remainder of the breakfast sandwiches into the trash can every day at the same time. Well, one day before I was about to "clock in", a very tempting idea came to my constantly never-satisfied mind..."why waste the sandwiches???" I wasn't thinking about feeding the homeless or those who really needed that food! I was thinking about myself. Of course! So I quickly grabbed every sandwich I could spot inside the trash can behind the counter. They were still wrapped after all. Delicious breakfast goodies with sausages or cheese-yum!?? No, I couldn't resist it! So I took as many as I could grab and quickly placed them between my stomach and the waistband of my black work pants. Then I made a run for the bathroom.....I was so excited! It was as if I had won the lottery (the "clogged artery lottery" that is)! I literally sat on a bathroom stall with door locked and devoured EVERY sandwich I had "scored" as if it was my last meal for 40 days and 40 nights. Wow, I never realized just what I was doing to myself back then, and I'm so glad I've started to undo that damage. And even though I haven't been to that restaurant for years, I still tend to roll the car window down and inhale deeply as I drive past!! Something about that smell that gets me every time. Once it hits your nostrils man it's crazy!! Just remember that some of you reading this will know exactly what I'm talking about and some of you may not. To those of you that relate to my stories you have to understand that you can pull yourself out of this hole. It takes practice and time and distractions to do so but you can. For those of you that have truly no clue..your day will soon come!

* * *

Fat confessional #15:

(Florida)

I live in Florida, land of sand, surf, sun and BATHING SUITS!!!!!!!!!!!!!! AHHHHHHHHHHH! For an over 300-pound, 16 year old brunette, the thought always sent shocks down my spine!! But my optimistic mom had spent like 90 something dollars to buy me a Brand-name bathing suit which promised support for my Size E boobs...I repeat…SIZE E!! (note: they are not size E anymore!) The bathing suit was a pretty bright blue and I was desperate for it to not only fit but for it to look nice. I tried it on and to my surprise it was extremely "supportive" for "the girls" and didn't cut into my cottage cheesy thighs, so now I was off to the beach!! Swimming, floating, I love it all and couldn't wait to hit the beach near my house. After spending time there, however, I'd had enough and was ready to head out of the water and home to my couch (of course). I waded out of the water, my eyes on the sand and seagulls. Nothing else intruded on my beach vibe. The ocean breeze caused me to shiver, and I suddenly realized why I was shivering when I noticed, in one of those slow motion experiences, that there was a reason, a real not-so-good REASON that caused everyone to stare. Yes, we all know Janet Jackson had a "nip slip" at that Superbowl and the internet's filled with stories of other celebrities who have experienced the same thing. But did Janet ever have the entire top half of her bathing suit fall open to the world? Did the straps of her suit ever rip off due to the amount of weight they had to hold up? Did she ever flash the entire public beach? Wait no... that was me! Not Janet! Holy moly, and I wasn't even a mermaid!!!!!!!!!

Fat confessional #16:

(swiss cheese pants)

SWISS CHEESE... not talking about eating it of course. I'm talking about being over 300 pounds with huge thunder thighs rubbing together so much that my pants would then take on the likeness of Swiss cheese-worn-away places and holes everywhere. When I was in my early 20's I waited tables. You run your butt off when you do that (at least I did) and I remember having to buy new work pants constantly because of my freshly made "holes". So I decided, why not make a contraption to prevent this from happening and save a few bucks?!! And I did! My contraption consisted of extremely large Feminine Pads and tape...You figure it out! Hey whatever! It worked! I helped keep that brand of "feminine napkins" in business, ok?! How's that for a personal confessional? Now the only holes I'm making are the extra loops on my belt to accommodate my ever -shrinking waist!!

*　*　*

Fat confessional #17:

(change sucks)

Found this today and it really is so true!!!! I was queen of comfort..comfort foods...comfort on the couch..routine routine routine. I still have to remind myself that I need to make changes if I want to keep getting results. Change is good though always scary..if you're on your journey or wanting to start it just remember to make small changes every couple of weeks. If you don't you will stall out and not to mention get bored. When exercise and fitness get boring we tend to slack off..and when we slack off..well you know what happens. DUM DUM DUM weight gain!!!!! So if you've been sticking to the same routine for a while now..be brave be daring be challenged! But just do not give up!!! This whole weight loss thing is so damn hard. It takes a STRONG person to win the battle. Just as in a real war you send your best people to the front of the line. If you don't send your best people then you lose the war. If you send people that think they are ready and they aren't you will lose anyways. Many of us never know if we're ready until WE ARE READY. You will know you are truly ready when those feelings hit you!!

* * *

Fat confessional #18:

(blame)

Growing up my parents would sometimes make small comments about my weight. Nothing horrible but noticeable enough. They definitely knew I had weight issues and sometimes reminded me of it daily. Especially once my room started smelling like stale food and I kept asking them what we were having for dinner the night before. But that's what food addiction does to people..it consumes you and envelopes your life with all of its icky forbidden goodness. You can blame your friends, family and any the latest flavored milkshake but you are to blame..and only you can get yourself out of this.

*   *   *

Fat confessional #19:

(treadmill bandit)

At one point, I had admitted to my parents, way back when at the ripe old age of 15, that I was unhappy with my weight and how I looked. So my mom suggested I try the treadmill she used. It was sitting off to the side of our living room and I decided to give it a try...After five minutes of walking on it, however, I decided I detested that thing, but couldn't bring myself to share the happy news with my family. And every day after I came home from school, I'd go into my living room (which was on the opposite side of the house from the kitchen hangout area) and I would turn on the treadmill and "workout". My workout consisted of sitting comfortably on the couch and lifting up the remote control, using it to search frantically for a rerun of "90210" or "Saved By The Bell"(Zac was sooo cute!). As I worked the remote and sat on the couch, the good ol' treadmill was a- chugging along- all by itself!! Every now and then I would walk over to it and bang my shoe on it to really make it sound as if I was "going hard" at exercising! Yeah, those were the days! And I still don't think I've ever admitted to my parents that my exercise sessions were anything but! Haha!

*　　*　　*

Fat confessional #20:

(jealousy doesn't become her)

I wish I had that..I wish I looked like her..must be nice to be that beautiful. That was me never ever loving myself and living with such bitter jealousy over almost every chick I saw. Well she's smaller than you Caitlin of course you're jealous over her. My jealousy would then turn into a massive bitchy attitude and I began treating people badly that didn't deserve it just because I was JEALOUS. Well envy did not suit me well at all and when I finally figured out this whole weight loss thing I thought to myself..if you aren't happy about yourself do something. I have the power to control my eating..I have the power to control how long I choose to dwell on the couch so why don't I?? It's not like wishing to lose weight and actually doing it is an unattainable dream..because it's not!! It just takes a special person to accomplish a tremendous amount of weight loss..I cannot begin to tell you just how many blisters I have counted on my toes and ankles..the number of band aids I have used is endless..the tired cranky mornings when I didn't want to get out of bed and chose to anyway..the no's to the second helpings when I really wanted to bury my face in the plate and pretend I was trying out for the Man VS Food reality tv show. The smell of popcorn tickling my nostrils at the movie theater while I ate carrot sticks instead. Knowing that this would be my job day in and day out for as long as it took and even when hitting wall after damn wall that I would reach that finish line one day. No amount of jealousy/envy or wishing you had someone elses life is going to change yours at all..you have the power to change your life. Do it already and stop wishing you were someone else.

* * *

Fat confessional #21:

(food thief)

If you knew me personally way back—back when I and my pre-teen girl friends would have sleepovers –you remember those, don't you?? Sleepovers? SO FUN! Complete with pillow fights, "makeovers", staying up all night long telling scary stories or talking about your "secret not-so-secret crush" at school and staging New Kids on the Blocks sing-a-longs; watching spooky movies that you were afraid of but wouldn't tell your friends that you were! Ahh, those were the days weren't they? If you were one of my teen friends and if that was your house I was crashed out on in the living room or bedroom then…I probably owe you and your family an apology! A big one, in fact!! So here goes:

I'm sorry! Sorry that I waited until everyone-all my friends at the party –was asleep. Sorry that I went tip toeing down the halls of a home I wasn't familiar with, banging my toe and bumping into numerous walls on my trek in the night. Why was I wandering around when I should have been crashed and asleep? The reason is that I had to find your kitchen in the dark-I had to discover what was inside that refrigerator in the kitchen. I'm sorry that I would slip so quietly into your hallway with all my thoughts focusing on one thing- eating what was in your fridge when you weren't around to see. When you invited me over to spend the night, I swear that those were not my intentions...it's not like I sat there and thought, "Hmmm, if I sleep at so and so's house I can devour all her food!! It's just that, well, my beast of a stomach was hungry and I had to satisfy the beast. The beast and the appetite! Your fridge was the way I chose to do so. It was always the best foods...the ones I didn't have at home that were kept away from me....because my family knew of my food addictions. They tried to help me stop by hiding any good treats from me....But IN YOUR HOUSE...IT WAS GAME ON!! Mac 'n cheese? Or maybe delicious leftover Lasagna?? CAKE? DID SOMEONE SAY CAKE? Or chocolate chip cookies??? I swear I ate as much as I could

23

without it being obvious. A spoonful of this and a forkful of that…you'd never know! And guess what?? Your mom does cook the best spaghetti ever!! You really weren't kidding! So to all of you out there whose house I ever stayed at for a sleepover, I am truly, dreadfully sorry for trying to (not purposefully) eat you out of house and home! I hope you can forgive me!!!!

*   *   *

Fat confessional #22:

(the little things)

OUT OF BREATH…miserable… constantly pulling at my clothes…looking in the mirror...eyes on the ground...yeah, that was life for me. Sweating constantly, no matter if it was winter or summer...yep, that was my story also! When something as simple as tying my shoes actually took my breath away, you would think that would've been my wakeup call!! But it wasn't. Instead I thought of new ways to put my shoes on without having to bend over, and tie the laces together which really only takes 3 seconds, but to me it was an eternity. Instead I would "side tie" the laces or tie them and manage to shove them on while standing and holding on to my living room wall and pray that my swollen fat feet would somehow get inside those shoes. Oh, the things that skinny people do daily and take for granted! Things that are so simple and easy and yet back then were the biggest obstacles in my life. Then, getting in and out of a car took at least 3 minutes longer than it should have. Struggling with the seat belt or the fact that I couldn't even use one, made a car trip nothing but a hassle. What would the traffic cop say if I tried to explain my fat situation when he pulled me over for a "click it or ticket?" "Sorry officer! I'm too fat!! Can't squeeze into the seat belt!" Would that work? Adjusting my steering wheel to make room for my enormous thunder thighs...or how about walking like a penguin to prevent those thighs from rubbing together. Or daring myself to wear shorts and then having to adjust them all day long as they rode up the inside of my legs...yeah, that's attractive! Way back when walking ten feet would make me feel like fainting… or suffering in the Florida heat that would chase me inside all summer long. Just looking back at all the things that we as large people had to adjust to, simply to be able to do daily activities, saddens me. So much time wasted, so much worry. So many amazing things missed. So much bullying and being treated like you're invisible, or not invisible enough, by people you're dying to get to know. It's so not worth it, people!

Honestly, is that 3rd slice of pizza worth all that to you? Or what about that second piece of cake? What about your kids? Are they on the same path I was?? Change it before it gets worse. Looking back I wish I had listened and learned sooner…learned that one day this girl would pretty much kill it. That one day this girl would be writing a book about her struggles or get featured on a weight loss site. That one day this girl would be getting certified to be a personal trainer. That one day this girl would look in the mirror naked and say: "Yeah, I have some cellulite and some loose skin but I worked hard, and I love myself, no matter what!"

* * *

Fat Confessional #23:

(music feeds my soul)

Just created a new playlist for weight lifting and one for cardio..i do this whenever i tend to get bored. Music honestly changes everything for me. Its funny how I love classic rock so very much but I can't stand working out to it. I find that I love rap when lifting and high speed techno when Im running..if you're getting bored with something change it..and that includes your tunes! Also buying cute new workout clothes helps...ALOT! They are now consuming my closet and I have more active wear than jeans..never thought I'd see that day coming! Reading some entries on my blog makes me laugh because I get as excited about reading them now as I did back when my life was ruled by food. It truly was all I thought about. Thank god it isn't that way now. I would miss way too much!

Fat confessional #24:

(STUCK)

STUCK!!!!!!!!! Yeah I said it…stuck! That was me, you know, the big fat girl over 300 pounds constantly getting stuck in things that I desperately needed help to get out of. The first time I really got stuck I was about 12 years old and attending a Catholic school in the next town over from my home in upstate New York. This first episode of being stuck was between me, my desk, and my trapper keeper notebook (YOU HAVE TO REMEMBER THOSE!). It doesn't sound too bad does it? It was. I can tell you that much because something very close to me got caught in my trapper keeper notebook. It was my belly fat!

There it is! It got caught in my trapper keeper. Please DO NOT ASK ME HOW! And it was all I could do not to scream for help in the middle of my classroom. After a minute of extreme panic, thankfully I managed to get free...but wait, there's more!!!

Yes, I was stuck yet again! Same age, same school, but this time it was on gym day. Oh lovely gym day!! My favorite day at school- YUCK!!! Fat girls do not like GYM DAY! Especially when they have to wear a gym sweat suit that makes them look like a big beached whale. My gym outfit was white of course! You get the picture! I swear GYM day was once a week and I almost always fibbed and told my parents or teachers that I had cramps and couldn't get to school that day. But nothing worked and I almost always had to go anyway! Well, I went to school with dread one day, just knowing I would have to exercise- OMG PLEASE NO. NOT THAT!!!!! It had rained the night before, you see, but despite that, our gym teacher decided, "Oohh lets go play volley ball outside, class!" With the rainy day and all, why she made that choice I'll never know! Regretfully I walked down the hill towards the volleyball net and the game got started. I dreaded the ball coming my way (prayed that it wouldn't). But of course it did. The most popular girl in my class spiked it my way and I thought, "Ok, here's my chance to fit in! If only I was good at volleyball, then they would like me!" (YEAHHHH SURE!). I dived for that ball with all my flab just flapping in the wind and then, "Bam!" I fell –HARD! Face first or shall I say, "face- planted"- right down, slipping and slopping, in a big puddle...a muddy hot mess of a puddle. Needless to say everyone laughed in uproar! Because big fat Caitlin got stuck in the mud and now she was covered from head to toe in the sloppy mess! What a sight! Fun and Games! Well, of course the school had no replacement for my mud-encrusted gym suit in my huge size there at the school, so I remained in them, waiting while my mom drove the longest 20 minutes ever to pick me up. Yeah, that was really fun. Especially fun when I dragged myself, the "Queen of SLIME", up the hill from the volleyball area, only to have the REST of the students in the entire school watch me from all the class windows that faced the hill. The whole school saw me, not just my own class! I still see that hill, that school, and the mud, in my dreams! Or nightmares!!

But wait! There's more! How about the time I went jet skiing (yeah, that was really out of my comfort zone) with two of my friends from high school and we hit a wave, a big wave! I flew off the back and got stuck literally directly underneath the jet ski! I tried with all my might to get back up, pulling and slipping on the wet surface, but my enormous chest (E CUPS Mind you!) were lodged underneath the jet ski so it took about 20 minutes and 2 people to help me back on top. That was also fun! And I've gotten stuck in so many turnstiles I cannot even count them (you know, as you're heading into those amusement parks). Oh, and speaking of amusement parks, have you ever been stuck on a roller coaster ride? Or a seat on an airplane?? I have been stuck at different times over the years on all these things, but you know what??? Finally, I got tired of being stuck!! Really sick and tired of that! So I put my big girl pants on (not that muddy white gym suit!) and worked my butt off and I'm proud to say I will never be stuck again. Thank you, goodnight!!

*   *   *

Fat confessional #25:

(AHA MOMENT)

I marked my calendar! Tomorrow is my "anniversary" -my anniversary of the first day I started eating healthy and working out... I decided to share a confessional that may not be as funny as the others, but it's honest and personal and you need to hear it!! Most of you know my story of losing over 150 lbs on my own without any surgeries or gimmicks! But do you know my AHA moment??

Well if you do, tough luck, you're gonna hear it again! In my early twenties, I was a waitress and was pretty darn good at it. In fact I had many regular customers/families that would come in to that local eatery. They would sit and wait until a table was open in my section. Sometimes my good friends would come in and try to get free food, and other times I was stuck waiting on people I didn't care for. That, and many other things, comes with the job!

A friend of mine happened to come in for lunch one day. I hadn't seen her in two years. I recognized her right away and was so excited to see her, but I'll never forget the look in her eye when she saw me. My friend looked shocked and almost a little embarrassed when she saw me headed her way. I went over to the table, spoke with her, asking how her life was, making small talk. She stood up and said, "OH MY GOD HOW FAR ALONG ARE YOU?????" Megaphone-loud, her voice boomed throughout the room, and that entire restaurant had heard every darn syllable that came out. Of course my face was burning hot red

I was so horribly humiliated. I thought in a quick second that maybe I should lie, but decided to downplay it, telling her she was mistaken. Indeed, I was not with child! She quickly apologized, of course, but the damage was done. Or maybe I should say the blessing, not the damage, had begun?

That day forever changed my entire world. Not that night though, not yet! I went home, cried myself into exhaustion. I sent for my comforts: I drank a gallon of milk and ate the cookies I always had nearby.   And the very next day I decided that enough was enough. I was sick and tired of the endless embarrassment, the humiliation, the clumsy episodes and false pregnancy reports! I was tired of wearing maternity clothes instead of regular things. Above all, I was simply TIRED OF STUFFING MY FACE and never being satisfied! So from that point, I "moved on" in my thinking and changed my entire attitude and life... And for the record, I will be forever grateful to my friend for her role in my turnaround. Because while it was horrible to hear and so humiliating at the time...and yet, her comment saved my life in the end. So, Happy Anniversary to me!!!

*   *   *

Fat confessional #26:

(sweaty hot mess)

Well, it's almost that time of year again folks…
well, at least down here in Florida it is. School
starts August 19th for us this year...and I was
thinking about it today as we approach the" Tax-
free shopping" weekend here in our county.
Thinking how excited I am to save a little bit on
some new clothes, since I'm blowing through sizes
fast enough (NOT COMPLAINING FOLKS).
But remembering just how much I HATED THIS
TIME OF YEAR GROWING UP...even though
It was always something I still looked forward to
year after year, no idea why, because by the end of
each shopping trip, I was crying my head off when
no one was around, and craving some chicken
nuggets for comfort... but yet, year after year, age
10, age 11, age 13… I still managed to be so
excited to go "SCHOOL SHOPPING" anyway!
(That's what we called "clothes shopping" for the
Daley kids before school started each year). But,
man oh man, did it suck for me. What was I so

unhappy about? Well, it hurt me that at age 12, I was 165 pounds and change. Funny that now, at age 33, and all grown up, I weigh less than that now! But picture this: Braces, DOUBLE D'S...yeah, they eventually bumped up to an "E", but thankfully, at age 12, God had only blessed me with double D's.(ONLY!) I've always had a small waist but an enormous caboose and thunder thighs galore. So you can imagine how tough it was for my poor mom to find clothes for me. I still remember her furrowed brow and worried looks! Because she had no flipping idea how she was going to get her daughter dressed for school. Funny thing is, since I went to a catholic school and we wore uniforms... pleated skirts to my knees, not looking at all fashionable like Britney Spears with her pleated minis!! But my mom forged onward with the whole school shopping thing because, what the heck! I couldn't wear pleated skirts all year round!?!? "Spandex" of course was in during this time and it was my BFF...WE WERE "TIGHT" BFFs though! Really tight, especially in the love handle area!! But, thanks to extremely long tee's that went down past my knees, I was covered up! Yep, I did that. But I still remember my mom taking me to women's sections- I was always confused as to why we would have to shop there. Why not shop in the

"COOL clothes " junior's area like everyone else? No, too bad, I couldn't get into the cool stuff. They didn't make the cool clothes in my size-not even close! I couldn't ever look like the rest of the girls and I used to get so upset about it. And as much as trying on clothes sucked-the worst thing was seeing them on my body in the mirror. Worst thing ever! Yep, it was all I could do to wait and get home afterward, before hobbling out of that mini -van and running, well not running, because let's face it, I didn't run back then...but yeah, hobbling up the steps to my bedroom and stuffing my face with the cream-filled cakes I had hidden in my closet and in other assorted areas of my bedroom.

Which begs the question: Why do people do this???? Why? If they know they are miserable and very, very out of shape, do they continue to eat junk and remain sedentary?? Why, why do we do this?!?! I ask myself that all the time, and each time, I come up with different answers all the time. But honestly, the bottom line is...change sucks! That's it! It's hard to change, to get out of that sleepy zone. No one likes it, and if you do change well, then you need to teach me to like change too! Routine has always been a best friend of mine...also fear and failure, being afraid of failing and yet failing because I was afraid all the time. I mean really, people!!!!!! You would think that after having to lie down on my pink canopy bed back in my upstate NY bedroom, so I could struggle with my zipper so much that my fingers would bleed, would've been my sign… THERE'S YOUR SIGN! Really!?!? Nope that wasn't it; it didn't happen for me then! And who would've thought that over 10 years later, I would finally get smacked in the face with it. It took too much to get me to that place!! Way too much!! It took years of being bullied; it took being treated like nothing, like an object of disgust by almost every boyfriend. It took not being able to buckle my seat belt or being able to tie my own shoes...it took me to practically eating my parents out of house and home, and what about those thousands of ants crawling on the dishes I'd hidden under my bed...It took heart palpitations...and swimsuit season, or the FAT PIG PICTURES taped to my locker daily at school by my loving 6TH grade classmates; it took the awful teasing , and the hair pulling, and the people in cars shouting at me on the side of the road...it took someone calling me pregnant!!! Where is your bottom line? Where is your, "OK, THAT'S ENOUGH! WHEN WILL YOU GET THERE??" Don't wait 28 long years to finally start living like I did...because you never know what will happen today, tomorrow, next week, next year. DON"T WAIT! Don't wait to BE GREAT!

*　　*　　*

Fat confessional #27:

(Mean gym rats)

I'll never forget the day I finally decided to walk in and DO IT! Do what? Hit the gym that is. It only took me losing my first 100 pounds to finally get up enough GUTS to step a single toe in there. But it wasn't because of my fitness abilities...nah! Are you kiddin'?? I knew I wasn't the greatest, but it for sure wasn't that. And it wasn't the cost of the gym membership because that's just the price ya gotta pay to drop the weight. It wasn't the sweaty muscled guys in love with their own appearance in the mirrors of the smelly free weights area. What was I so scared of??? If it wasn't the muscled guys, or the prices, or the machines, what was it? It was "THE MEAN GIRLS" of course! Yep, THOSE mean girls. They literally scared the heck out of me without even saying a word to me. You know who I'm talking about-- those girls, the gorgeous ones who never had to work for it, who never had to bead up from a workout or get their nails broken on the weights. The girls that never had to work for anything at all. Yep, those are the girls who wear more makeup to the gym than Lady Gaga on tour. The ones who have the absolute hottest brand-name workout clothes that I have ever seen! Those are the girls that I so desperately wanted to be. THOSE MEAN GIRLS!! The girls who don't hit the gym to workout-ever! Those girls who go to get "hit on" by guys and hog all the machines that we real girls need more than they do! YES THEM! They kept me away from living healthy for 80 POUNDS of my life...And not to mention the fact that I still, even after losing my first 100 Pounds, felt intimidated by them. Even as I began to run faster than they did on the treadmills (which isn't hard to do lol.) But I still let them get to me. They didn't even know me, nor care to of course, and I'm sure the last thing they were thinking of was of me...the girl wearing nasty stained clothes with holes in them, struggling to run with 3 sports bras on...nah, it was never about anything else but them. Fast forward to now...I see these mean girls in a totally different light. I see them as dying to be accepted. Craving male attention and wanting all eyes on them as they enter the room. Maybe they don't get enough attention at home and this is the one place where they do get noticed. Or maybe they see themselves being ugly and this one place, the gym, makes them feel beautiful. But I can tell you that I am one of those girls now! Minus the bitchy attitude...minus the perfect hair and bling accessories. Now I'm the girl getting the looks and the obvious stares cast in my direction. So when you see me heading into the gym looking all cute...please say "Hi" to me. Because I won't judge you... I will accept you for who you are. I will not judge you or make you feel like dirt. Because the only difference between me and the other pretty girls happens as I leave the gym! I leave it covered in big sweat! A big SWEATY MESS! No makeup, no perfect hair, and no fashion dream clothes! So don't —don't let people you don't know drag you down, nor people you do know, for that matter!! Don't be scared of your gym...embrace it and embrace the changes it will offer your mind and your body!! I promise you that walking out of those doors soaked in sweat will beat down every negative comment or stare that was thrown at you when you first walked in!

* * *

Fat confessional #28:

(lazy days)

You know that feeling you get when you come home from work and you're so tired and the couch looks SO darn comfortable and you just want to sit there for a minute, just a short minute!? And that one minute turns into 5 and that 5 minutes turns into 60 minutes and pretty soon you don't want to do anything else? I know you know that feeling. Well… SNAP OUT OF IT!!!!!!!!!! That was me today after I got home from work and I forced myself to hit the gym for Turbo class…and right about now I feel like a million bucks. A real million really sweaty bucks!!

* * *

Fat confessional #29:

(extracurricular activities)

Remember those "Extracurricular activities" that revolved around school when we were kids? You know by now that extracurricular activities were never my thing when I was fat...mainly because I preferred not to move or make the effort! But by second or third grade I decided to join the group after all. The group with the great COOKIES! Well now, that was something I could do. Why was that different? It was those cookies!!!! The wonderful cookies!! Sell cookies? Come on people, if I can eat them, I can sell them! I wasn't so much into all the other activities in the group, the badges and the camping out, etc. etc. But the cookies! That was the thing! So, I still remember the first time I laid my hungry eyes on those little boxes! That large, purple glossy- looking one with the golden name written all over it...the cookies inside-they looked amazing!! I had to get my hands on those! The chocolate minty ones... sorry, just not my thing...no, it was the purple box cookies that I loved best! Basically they had me at first box...or better yet, I fell in love after the first bite. This 9- year -old girl with the braces and weight problem had a new addiction. Oh boy! I knew right then and there that I would do anything to get my hands on those darn little cookies!!! I didn't care what it took! So I started with a new strategy this time! On that big order sheet I took home, I would change my parents' cookie selections by erasing the one or two boxes my mom had written, and I would write in a larger number of boxes instead! That way we "*Accidentally*" received way too many cookies. Oh no!! How did that happen!!? Well luckily, nobody cared! Or really noticed! And when the order arrived, I ran with them up to my room, hidden under my jacket like a lost puppy!! No wet nose and floppy ears here, just boxes-my boxes! And before I knew it, one box turned into two, then three, four… All stashed in random places around my pink flower wallpapered bedroom with the pretty canopy bed! Oh, the joys of my prized boxes!

* * *

Fat confessional #30:

(Girl Scout cookies)

Being a brownie had its perks for some but not me...I just wanted to EAT the brownie --not BE one! Well, maybe there were some perks to it after all! The camping trips that I found so boring, turned into a plus when everyone fell asleep at night. Everyone slept while I would: a. eat all the marshmallows from the "smores" we made earlier, or: b. sneak into lunch boxes and help myself! Yes, I admit it. And I never saw it as wrong then at all. Looking back now I realize how horrible that is and that right now in this world there's a little 9- year- old camper doing the same darn thing I did because she can't help herself!! Now, when I pass by the outdoor cookie stands every spring at the local stores and see the girls standing there so eager to sell… I chuckle to myself when I remember all the drama from back then. But I still move quickly through the entry doors to get away from the memories of those days! My memories of those attractive little boxes with their amazing goodies inside!! Yes, things have changed for me since then, and now I wonder what would happen if they sold carrot sticks and hummus instead??

* * *

Fat Confessional #31

(skinnies please listen)

If you've never been fat before in your life, then this one is for you...if you've never had more rolls on your stomach that your local grocery bakery department, then this one is for you… if you've never been too fat to bend over and tie your shoelaces, then this one is for you... And if you've never sneaked food into a closet to eat it at midnight then this one is for you too!! What am I talking about?? Well, I'm talking about the way society treats fat people of course! You would think that in this day and age, when 1 in 3 Americans are considered obese, that it wouldn't be a big deal to see a large person in public...but that's just not the case. I'm not at all saying people should ignore their health and embrace the weight... I'm just saying you would think people would be a little nicer to those that aren't blessed enough to live in mini- skirts and string jeans! If you see someone out there who is struggling, then instead of pointing and laughing at them with your friends, or ignoring them, why not reach out? Why not make it your goal to help that person? Are you scared someone will make fun of you for friending a fattie? If you don't understand what this confessional is about, well let me break it down for you. Here goes: One of my favorite movies is "Pretty Woman". I'm sure you all know the story line: Julia Roberts is a "lady of the night" who meets a glamorous Richard Gere, and they fall in love. Great Hollywood ending! But there is a scene in that movie that totally stands out for me and honestly gives me flashbacks of my former fat self. In the movie after Julia meets Richard, he hands her a stack of cash and tells her to hit up Rodeo drive for some snazzy threads. Julia then walks into a boutique in her "evening" clothes (blue mini skirt...thigh highs...you remember!) and she is ignored; treated like gutter trash and refused service. All because of her clothes and appearance. Later on, Julia returns in her classy dress and tells the sales woman what a big mistake she's made! Since she works on commission! Julia won the battle! And it pretty much shows how Karma really is a bitch! I cannot begin to tell you just how many times this has happened to me at many a mall store or clothing boutique-unless it had the "Plus Sized" label and "Plus sized" women's clothes! People can be downright hateful because of how you look on the outside. But if they ever took the time to really get to know me, then who would they know? Well, they'd find a girl from New York that does a kick -ass Drew Barrymore impression, and who can listen to your problems for hours and make you laugh for even longer than that. It's amazing how I'm treated so differently compared to the ME of before. I'm still the same ME...I still do those silly impressions and I still promise to try and make you laugh for hours. There's just LESS of me now! Less skin, less blubber. So the next time you point and laugh at someone or ignore them instead of smiling and holding the door for them or whatever...remember who they are, a human being who could use a friendly greeting! The media are full of sad stories about kids who are bullied and abused at school. If every student reached out and became a friend to others, then those stories would change! So do your part: Show interest in another human being. Because you never know just what treasure lies underneath. Just like you never knew what I was hiding inside: beauty on the inside and outside too! I'm grateful that I have completely changed my life for the better, but all I've done really, is lose a lot of weight...which any of you can do. But I'm still the same funny Cait after all!

*   *   *

Fat Confessional #32

(skeletons in closet)

Tonight my confessional is a little different...But I feel I just had to go to the darkest place and open it up really wide...and let everyone in to see. Why? Because sometimes I have to defend myself about losing all this weight. Why? Because it's amazing that I've lost so much...because no one thinks it can be done without the help of surgery or diet pills and starvation. But I chose a different route… I chose to do it on my own. With nobody helping me (well, except for my family cheering me on! They tried to help, but it had to come from me, after all!). I chose to do it the smart way...to work my butt off for over 4 years now! Yeah, it took me longer than it would've if I could've afforded a trainer and it took me longer than it would've if I had been a contestant on a reality show trying to win big money for my weight loss. It took longer than it would have if I had gone under the knife and risked my life for beauty. But I don't flipping care. For every ounce of sweat, for every ounce of hating to lace up my shoes, for every ounce of missing bad food and for every ounce of negativity, I chose to push on harder and harder! I chose to drown in my sweat...I chose to learn to live with sore muscles...and I chose to learn to say NO!" No to those endless "second" helpings... I chose to get up at the crack of dawn while everyone else was asleep. I chose to ignore temptations or say no to birthday invites and dinner dates for fear of overeating! I chose to make sacrifices in my life that really aren't sacrifices...I chose to give up WANTS and replace them with NEEDS instead. If someone asked me if I woke up tomorrow as the old Caitlin-would I do it all over again?? ABSOLUTELY I would! Definitely!! I've lived on that side of the fence...lived on that side and was always looking past the wooden posts...nose peeking over the fence desperately trying to get over it. Trying to get over that fence and live on the happier side of life. I would absolutely do it all over again if I had to...because it's changed my life that much. I've never felt better about myself in my entire life. I type it out and look at it in amazement and really mean it...I've never thought I looked better. Though I never did think I would love myself. The funny girl that cracked jokes about herself hated who she was so much it's not even funny- wasn't funny then or now! And what about now? Well, I wouldn't trade places with anyone, that's NOW! Because who I am is amazing!! So tonight, I share with you my deepest, darkest part of me...that indeed I did not go "under the knife"...that indeed I chose to kick ass and sweat instead! Now consider these my new "before" pics...because I'm getting ALL THIS off...the healthy happy way!! Just watch me!

*   *   *

Fat confessional #33:

(dirty mouth)

(*Warning: this next confessional contains a bad word!*)
I'm sure many of you can remember the first time
you said a bad word in front of your parents...or
maybe you can't but I sure can!..I remember it like
it was last week! Why would saying a curse word
be so significant to me???? Well, if you were raised
in a catholic family (by a Southern Mom!) it would
rock the heck out of your world also. Growing up
as a kid, the bad words we knew were "shut up"
and calling someone "stupid"! Haha. Seems so
innocent now compared to all the stuff coming out
of people's mouths in this day and age (mine
included!)...But the funny thing about my bad word
is that it involved something that's really good:
food! Yeah- that's a shocker right?? A former fat
chick upset about food? NOOOOO!! Yeah! Of
course! So here we go! The year was 1991...I
remember the year because my little brother was
due to come into the world any day back then, and
I was super excited to welcome him into the world
with my other siblings. But I also remember the
year because of where my bad word took place. I'll
give you a hint, follow along... it was in a dark
place. A very dark place! It smelled absolutely
amazing and the seats had cup holders!!! The seats
were ok but the screen...man oh man --was it huge
and we were so close!!! Where was I? At the
movie theater of course!! I'll never forget the day!

It was so cold outside that February! Being in such a large family (5 kids total) we rarely went to the movies, but watched the VHS ones (remember?) at home! So this was a huge and very special treat! What movie did we see? HOME ALONE!!!! Hello! It was just past Christmas time and it was cold and it was 1991!!! So we were all excited for the movie to begin and dad had just brought us all some popcorn and sodas-yum! The ultimate treat! The movie began and we were all quietly munching away when it happened...(DUM- DUM- DUM...) I dropped my popcorn bag and watched every buttery kernel fall to the floor that already looked like it had never made friends with a broom and mop! Every luscious buttery kernel! It was in slow motion and I could hear myself say THAT word...I felt as if I were watching myself say it! Here it comes: "OH S...t!!! "! Really? I honestly have no idea how I learned the phrase! Not from my parents, who were very good about never cursing around us. Whatever... it came out! And it came out loud and cruel sounding too! I was so pissed off that I had dropped all of the amazing movie theater popcorn (of course, there's no other popcorn like movie popcorn!!) all over the place!!! After uttering those words, I was scared to death...scared to look up at my mom and dad because I knew what was coming. They were shocked not only because I said but because of what drove me to say it. FOOD!!!!!!!!!!!!! BLEH FOOD!!! All that upset over-- FOOD??? How that four-letter-word, the REAL "bad word", ruled my world! How it ruined so much of my life at such a very young age. Do not, I repeat, do not let it ruin yours! Do not let food control you or change you, or make you say and do bad things! Do I have a "sailor mouth" now??...Honestly, yes I do sometimes! But it's not because of that four-letter-word anymore!!!   It's because of that OTHER FOUR LETTER WORD: DIET! Yes, Diet can be a FOUR LETTER WORD-when it's not healthy and clean! So make that choice to clear up your health and your habits! You will eventually clean all other areas of your life as well!

*   *   *

Fat Confessional #34

(fat suit)

I can't quite remember when my "fat suit" started showing...after all; I wore it for over 25 years! I wasn't fat as a baby, just cute, according to my mom, who says I did have the cutest little chub cheeks ever! But I wasn't fat! I wasn't even fat by age 8! Looking back through old pictures and albums of the family, I see that I wasn't the tiniest thing but I certainly wasn't fat. So when did the fat suit come? Sometimes I feel like I just woke up one day and I was obese. How could that be? After all, I didn't get that way on my own account! It HAD to be somebody else who forced me to eat that 5th piece of cake back then!! Man, cake! (I could sure go for some of that great Buttercream frosting right about now.) And it had to be a bad nightmare that I would clean off my plate and then, when nobody else was looking, I'd take extra servings. Or maybe it was after all the dinner dishes got washed and put away, and I knew my parents were outside or elsewhere in the house, or watching tv in another room away from the kitchen area. Maybe it was then...then, I could, and did, sneak quietly back into the kitchen into the leftovers on the stove and happily grab a few more forkfuls of pasta, or stew, or whatever! I always ate like I it was my last meal! I always ate like I was headed off to "Survivor" where I had to compete to win food. Hunger games I could relate to! I guess you could say my whole young life was a "Hunger Game!"

Nah, that isn't how I got fat-- But yet, it is. That IS how it happened! That is how it went down... and that is how my life went from being the girl with the big green eyes and dimples to being the chick with dimples on her upper thighs. I'm not saying this is how some of you got that way; what I'm saying is this is how I changed my life. I changed the plan God made for me at such a young age. I mean, really, I weighed 160 pounds at age 9!! Yes, I did! I officially weigh LESS than I did at age 9 - NOW! Insane!! But when you celebrate with food, grieve with food, and practically make out with your dinner plate well... HELLO! It's bound to happen!

*   *   *

Fat Confessional #35:

(honey hide the sweets)

My parents did everything they could to try and help me! There was the "hiding the sweets" strategy, but I'm telling you I could find a chocolate chip cookie better than I could find Waldo in that book. I was the "Nancy Drew of foodery". I could find it anywhere!! Not that it's something good that I would even brag about. By the time I realized the fat suit was enormous, I had already given up...felt that it was too late for me. The nail had been placed on the coffin and hammered in, so to speak. The fat lady had sung...literally! In my teens I would lose 5 pounds, then gain 10, lose 20 pounds, gain 15...A constant roller coaster of binge eating and hating life...a merry go round that had no "off" switch.

Fat Confessional : #36

(quitter)

I was always a starter...starting was never a problem for me like it is for some, but man could I QUIT!! I was a champion QUITTER! I could quit better than anyone I knew!! I would work out with such passion and intensity and then immediately drink down a gallon of milk while eating those brownies. Does anyone know the term "sugar addiction"!!? That's it people! I would practically exercise with food in my hands. Really? Yes, it's the truth! I had no idea that I would have to eat healthy AND exercise. Nobody had told me they go hand in hand-or if they did, I wasn't listening! Nobody told me about that starvation feeling you get when you first start out-that panicky kind of thought: "I'm starving!" Nobody told me I had to learn to say no and push plates away. (Well, they did, but I ignored them!) If I didn't listen, it was because it was my job to discover all that on my own. They couldn't do it for me! To those of you out there who were just like me...starting and quitting-starting and quitting: How do you expect to get anywhere with the life you want? If losing weight was easy we would all be fit. Well it's true!!! Pay attention to your body, treat your body as a temple, love your body the way you see fit. If you think your body deserves 2 bagels slathered in Philadelphia cream cheese, then by all means go for it. But do not complain later when your pants are tighter than tight, and then say: "Wow, how did I gain those 5 pounds!!??!??!" You know how you gained the 5 pounds...just like I did. I might've changed my life plan at a young age...I might've placed the nail on the coffin and hammered it in. But I can tell you one thing...I kicked the crap out of that old life and gained such an amazing one...hard work...tears...determination...sweat...courage...perseverance! Heck, basically I did this as a second job. Losing weight and getting healthy are a second job to me. Because it's a lifestyle change. You can't celebrate after losing 50 pounds, think you're healed and walk away from the process...doesn't happen that way! I've done that! It comes creeping back! So start and do not quit...change your life plan now!

*　*　*

Fat Confessional #37:

(Fast food to magazines)

From Fast Food...to Magazines...This is a big one people -so pay attention!! 90% of you do not know me personally....although you may feel like you do! All you know is what I tell you and share with you, but you don't know me other than that. So let me remind you of a few things the next time you stick your nose in the fridge looking for a third helping of lasagna! This doesn't just happen overnight. To lose the weight you need to WORK at it. You can't lose it and quit...says who? ME! You know why? Because it doesn't work that way! How do I know? BECAUSE I QUIT! I started in 2008 and after two years I gave up. Got burned out. Threw in the towel...the sweaty towel. I was so tired of exercising and eating healthy!! I thought, "That's it, the heck with this...I've lost all my weight and now I'm cured!! Now I'm disease-free and can eat whatever the heck I want and I do not need to run, or walk, or lift anymore either! Big mistake! And I kept on going down...and down to those fast food lines! 4 big burgers with cheese and a large order of fries, and there I sat in my old "grand am", hiding out, mired in grease and regret. Why did I do this-become my own worst enemy! And why did I choose to fail? Because it's easier to fail...because it's easier to quit and throw in the towel. Losing weight has been the toughest road I've ever been on...think "one -lane highway covered in ice tough" ...because that's what it is! Those burgers tasted good for 5 seconds and yet in that 5 seconds I had ruined my self esteem, my confidence and everything I had worked hard for! Two years shot…all my hopes completely crushed! Me alone with my miserable self and crying my eyes out.

Enough was enough!! So I got back on the weight loss wagon the very next day…vowing that I would never ever fall off it again! I was tired of being bruised and broken…tired of starting over and over again, and tired of doing so much damage to my body just by quitting. So what happens WHEN YOU START AND STOP? All the feelings that I mentioned before happen…hopelessness…hating yourself and everyone in your life…detesting your reflection in the mirror and crying from the pain of your thunder thighs rubbing together when you walk. You have your highs and your lows, but you have to KEEP ON GOING. You have it in you- just like I did and still do! If this was easy the world would look like those awesome movie stars! If this was easy there would be no such thing as high medical bills or kids getting fatter and fatter…there would be no such thing as empty calories, or hiding out in your car with 4 burgers, and not eating at the dinner table anymore with your family because you're "too busy"!

What happens WHEN YOU START AND KEEP GOING? You get to share your story with the world...and help others...you get to blog about it and start writing that book you always wanted to write! You get to run challenge groups and help others feel as good as you do now. Then, you get to study to be a certified personal trainer with NASM... But most importantly... you put yourself out there and you get a bite... a big bite… from SHAPE MAGAZINE! Suddenly, you see yourself featured in their November issue!! Yes, that's right: this chick that used to weigh over 300 pounds is going to be in a magazine! I've worked so hard for this and every day was worth it. Never, ever QUIT, never!! You can't know where your path will take you when you start- so keep going- and never quit!

*   *   *

Fat Confessional #38:

(full)

For those of you that have followed me from the very beginning, some of these may sound familiar...or maybe they just sound familiar because you yourself have done this! You yourself also had or still have a HUGE emotional eating issue that you have tried to hide for years but just cannot hide it any longer. But just what does emotional eating do to your body? Well, besides making you a mountain of over 300 pounds of flab like I was at one point in my life, what else does it do? It makes for a life of misery and regret. A life of negativity and dread. A life where no fork is left unturned. Who the heck even knows what it's like to be full? That was my state of mind...those were my thoughts. I'll never forget the fast food commercial where the people got excited that they screamed it from the top of their lungs! Why were they screaming? Because they felt FULL! That's a feeling I never knew in those days of fat in the fat suit I wore! Hunger pangs were my constant companions… I was never satisfied, ever! I only knew dirty size 28 jeans that I didn't wash ever because they shrunk in the wash and I needed them as loose as possible. I only knew what it looked to have 4 boobs because my bras were so damn tight they would cut my boobs in half and leave them spilling over so I always looked like I was blessed (or cursed) with 4 boobs, not 2…And there was that tugging! Always tugging down on my enormous Tee shirts and fat lady tops. If you know what that feeling is like, comment on this confessional!!! I only knew what red and chafed thighs were and that I would dump loads of powder on them to soothe them and hopefully (fingers crossed) prevent them from rubbing together while I waited on customers at work. Of course it never worked though!! I felt like I only knew what it was like to steal food out of every kitchen I came into contact with, whether it be at home, my parents' refrigerator, my jobs, my friends' houses...no kitchen was left unturned!!! No leftover lasagna untouched!! No icing left unlicked!! I occupied more drive thru windows at fast food joints than birthday parties, or proms, or dressing rooms!! No joke people!! I get it all the time... How hard it is for people to picture me as the fat funny chick-and I was always funny with people! I was the fat, funny chick that laughed at everything and cracked people up! My face to the world! Then I would put myself in my car sideways and struggle with wrapping a seat belt on and cry the whole way home.

* * *

Fat Confessional #39:

(pep talk)

I can't begin to tell you how much this journey to wellness sucked the minute I started at the gym. I'm not gonna lie- it wasn't pretty! There was a lot of crying, dry heaving from the work outs...and the starving!! No, I did not starve myself to get here, but when you go from consuming who knows how many gallons of milk daily and a large stuffed crust supreme from Pizza Hut by yourself...well, even taking a fraction of your daily intake out can leave you a little hungry!! It was an addiction and I was in rehab, with a long road ahead of me! I knew it would be tough...I knew I would fall down, I knew I would fail countless times. I just never knew I would pick myself back up once and for all and give my fat the middle finger and never say hello to it again! You've got it in you...that fight...that (good) hunger for a better life. Now get it!!!

*   *   *

Fat Confessional #40:

(don't hate)

Why do you workout so much? Why do you eat so healthy all the time? Why do you get excited to go to the gym? WHY, WHY, WHY!!!!!!!!!!!!! If I get asked these questions one more time...Yes I hear them on a daily basis!! At first I would always sit there and explain myself, as if being over 300-something pounds and not being that way anymore needed some sort of an explanation!! Really? But apparently in this day and age, it does. I work out because I do love it! I love what it has done for my self esteem, my confidence level, my life, my marriage, my friends…the list goes on and on! I eat healthy because it's the way God intended. Temptation from junk food gives a quick feel-good moment, but it only lasts a minute and… man does that feeling go away fast! And what's left? REGRET…MISERY…AND TIGHT JEANS! So, I eat healthy because I know I need to…I eat healthy because I enjoy it! Is it more expensive? Yup! It is!! And is having two gym memberships for myself expensive? Yup!! But I'm worth every penny spent. I'd rather use the hard- earned money I make on stuff like that…rather than hundreds of dollars on high blood pressure or diabetes meds later on down the road. So why do I get excited to workout?? Because I've worked my ass off for that good feeling I get! I have made this my "second "full time job. It's my priority. What other excuses do I hear?? Oh yeah, of course I get the… "well, you don't have kids yet, so you have the time for it, of course!" You think I wouldn't be working out if I had kids???? Try me! Because I would and when that happens, I will. YOU HAVE TO MAKE THE TIME FOR YOURSELF! So do not- I repeat- DO NOT take the easy road out!! I've taken it and always had to

U-TURN right back where I came from. Take the time... even if it's only 10 stinking minutes a day.

* * *

Fat confessional #41:

(not enough time?)

If you have time to read my posts...you can work out. Even if you don't have a feeling of respect for yourself! Even if you have no idea what it's like to actually, from the bottom of your heart, love yourself...like I do now! You will make the adjustments needed to live a fitter, healthier and longer life. Don't wait for Monday... man, I cannot tell you how many Mondays came and went and nothing happened! Oh, I can eat like crap this weekend because Monday is coming and then I am going to start my "diet" -EWW THAT WORD! But man oh man did I say it!! Well, take that out of your vocabulary because diets fail...diets (there's that four-letter-word again!) do not work for a year or a lifetime. I pray all the time and I am so eternally grateful for my wake up call, because what If I had never gotten it?? Where would I be right now?? Crying over a box of doughnuts??...yup!! Well that's it folks!! But wait...you've probably seen me in pics with friends and family members on my blog. Sometimes my little brother, who is all of 160 pounds, gets in a photo with me. But I realized one day that I have officially lost him! I HAVE OFFICIALLY LOST A PATRICK...I have lost my brother's weight- plus 22 pounds- from my body!! And I am so damn proud of it. This is why you take the road less traveled... this is why you do not quit ever!!!!!!!!

* * *

Fat Confessional #42

(Imposter)

IMPOSTER!!! I totally felt like an imposter yesterday when I was clothes shopping with my hubby! Why?? I felt like an imposter because I was trying on size 4 pants and size small tops...and they fit! I felt like an imposter so much so that I actually was in the "plus size" section before I realized I didn't need to be there anymore. You would think that by now I would get it... get that I've worked my ass off and deserve to be in the smaller section!! Get that I have soaked myself in sweat everyday for 4 years for this!! And get that not only have I accomplished dropping all this weight on my own-achieving a HUGE milestone for myself and many others along the way!! My Shape Magazine feature coming up in November still feels like a dream and I am dying to see that magazine arrive at my doorstep. Then, my personal training certification is almost complete, so I can help change others lives as well, and getting two legs into ONE of my old pair of jeans-no, I am NOT AN IMPOSTER! But the old, insecure Caitlin sometimes does tend to show herself from time to time… not as much as she used to… but she still can be a bother. So, as I started to head into the dressing room with the clothing, it was my husband who stopped me and asked, "Why do you have a medium and a large outfit?? You're a SMALL!!" Pinch me- I'm dreaming!!! I laughed at myself and went back for the smaller selections and I thought to myself, "No Caitlin, you don't have to hit that area of the store ever again! You don't have to worry about being called a cow anymore or that awful rubbing feeling from your enormous thighs! All you have to worry about now is upping your weights, staying on track... and paying it forward to help others get started on that path-- so they won't feel like imposters either!!!

*　　*　　*

Fat Confessional #43:

(you are what you eat)

You really are what you eat!!   Boy, am I living, freakin' proof of that... countless excuses, not to mention the countless lies I told to EVERYONE... even people I loved!!!   "How did you get so fat, Caitlin??"   Me? Really??   I have no idea because I barely eat...LIES ALL OF THEM!! I knew what I was doing. I knew which hand held the fork and which hand held the heaping cup of soda! I still remember my first taste of ANYTHING baked from the grocery store!   All those logo faces smiling on the fronts of the junk food boxes! Those little boxes that will forever ruin your life, your scale and your pants size.   But I had a SERIOUS ADDICTION to those little cakes you see waiting for you at the end of the aisle shelf! Anything with cream in it, or striped with vanilla and chocolate icing (here we go with cake again people)! If you have never heard of these delectable but dangerous treats... that's GOOD!! I wish I hadn't! I was in my teens the first time I had ever really laid eyes on those little boxes...the demon spawn of a treat! I was hooked at first bite...I was a junkie looking for a fix...a dog searching for his bone. And I found my bone in that white box with the delicious looking cakes inside! 12 of them to be exact; which I might add were all demolished in one sitting! One entire box of oatmeal pies- a dozen!! Grand total in calories 2040...fat calories are 720...not to mention all the other crap in there!! But I didn't care then about the numbers...instead I polished off an entire box of those goodies... EVERY SINGLE NIGHT!! I used to make my husband drive and get me boxes of them and soon he also had an addiction!! And why not? Misery loves company! I was eating them and they satisfied my sweet tooth and were cheap all at the same time. I used to stuff them in my purse and sneak them into the bathroom at work just like I did with basically everything else. "IF THEY DON'T SEE ME EATING IT, THAT MEANS I'M NOT!" I thought. I almost always went in that direction in my mind...if I'm not caught eating this stuff etc. etc ... Then, It never happened! What happens in Vegas stays in Vegas!

Yeah I'm sure it does... but what happens when that little cake box and all those hidden treats don't just stay hidden and locked away from the world. Nope, they reared their ugly face on my thighs...my ass...my stomach and that attractive triple chin I wore! It's such a shame that snacks like these are still sold and are STILL CHEAP!! Some families just don't think they have any other options but to purchase that junk! Instead, people, INVEST!! Invest in yourself --it is SO worth it!! Yeah, I know that Kale or broccoli doesn't taste like a delicious little cream cake! But man, does it look GOOD on my ass!!! So don't live in denial any longer-- you really are what you eat, and once again, I am proof of that! Eat junky crap and you will weigh over 300 pounds...eat healthy and you won't. It's that simple. Now put your forks down and move!

* * *

Fat Confessional #44:

(screw portion control)

PLEASE PASS ME SOME MORE!! Some more what??? FOOD!!!!!!!!!!!

Firsts...seconds...thirds...sometimes even fourths!!! I had a bottomless pit, not a stomach... a never ending appetite for every damn thing put in front of me. Portion control? What IN THE WORLD was THAT??? Chewing slowly? I think not!!! I remember once reading that for every bite of food, you should chew 20 times...20 TIMES!! When I read this, I was about halfway to my heaviest weight and I actually almost choked on my cookies as I ate and read the words...20 TIMES??????? NEVER!! And I was too rushed to actually take the time to enjoy my meals. I gobbled them fast and furious in the hopes that nobody knew just how many helpings I had consumed! I stuffed it down so quickly I couldn't even enjoy all the calories or the sugar that would eventually cling to my hips later on, anyway. I inhaled what was on my plate instead of eating it...never savored each bite...there was no time... I had to keep chomping and stuffing! It was in my mouth the second it was in my face. That's why it's so embarrassing to look back at old pics or old home videos of myself and truly SEE what eating ... JUST EATING... had done to my body...my mind...my self esteem and most of all my self control. Fitness and nutrition really and truly do go hand in hand and I don't care how long I spend working out!! If my eating sucks I will not look fit...it just sits there... right on my hips. As if seconds and thirds wasn't enough for this girl back then! I ate so quickly that an hour later I was starving all over again. Of course, it was because what I was consuming wasn't giving me what my poor big body needed... because it was all junk. Burger after burger, pizza slice after pizza slice, CAKE AFTER CAKE (WE ALL KNOW IT'S MY FAVE!)...washed down with gallons of milk downed in one day not by my family but by ME!! It's a wonder I'm still alive to tell this tale! I recently asked my mom a few weeks ago to tell me things I used to do when I was young-- as if I ever could forget--and she said to me, "THE MILK!! The milk was always gone!! ". She had always thought it was because she had five amazing kids who loved getting their calcium fix, but it wasn't... IT WAS ME-- ONLY ME!! The money my mom spent on milk back in the day just for my consumption...wow!!!! That Mindless Eating! If you haven't heard that term before, then you just did! Mindless eating was my middle name...hand to mouth, hand to mouth, staring at the TV for hours with those chips and dip, not even realizing just how much I had until my fingers hit the bottom of the bag! A second on my lips--forever on the hips! The saying is so true! Just like "you are what you eat" is true! Well, these hips don't lie now!! I'm a clean eating machine! Now I sit down and stare at my food for a minute...literally... and I look at what is on my plate and inhale the intoxicating scent. I truly make it an event. Then, I chew slowly… maybe not 20 chews per bite… BUT I'M WORKING ON IT, OK?!?! PAY ATTENTION to what you are PUTTING in your mouth... that is the secret. If you can conquer the battle with the kitchen you, my friends, can be on the right path! So I raise my fork with happiness and finally without GUILT, because I know that the food I'm about to dig it into-is EXACTLY what I should be eating!!

* * *

Fat Confessional #45:

(love thyself)

As I read through emails that I get from all the wonderful people who are following my page, I find a common theme among many of them. Quite simply, it's this: it's the lack of love they have for themselves! That's it! And I've been there, trust me... I never loved myself before... I didn't even like me. I couldn't stand the sight of myself! All those fat rolls, those stretch marks, all that cellulite, it never ended! My body looked like a road map!!!!! That's no lie! If you want to love yourself, you need to invest in yourself... you need to make the time... you need to eat healthy… you need to drink water… you need to give up bad addictions. Step-by-step! Once you can master all that you will finally see just how wonderful you really are!! Can it be overwhelming? Heck yes, it can be!! But if you want it so badly that you can taste it... you won't stop at anything! You will slip... you will fall… but you will overcome those tiny mistakes and celebrate your victories if you stick to it! Do I still have stretch marks?? YES! Do I still have cellulite?? YOU BET I DO! Is there loose skin here, there, and everywhere?? Just ask my hubby!! Yes, yes!! But do I finally love myself no matter what? Truthfully? I've never loved anybody more... and that's a good thing!

* * *

Fat Confessional #46:

(million dollars)

If somebody offered to pay me a million dollars to
get healthy over ten years ago, I would've
laughed… and of course, taken the bet! I mean
come on, who wouldn't have??? What I could do
with a million bucks? Well, let's see...pay off
debts/student loans…car… take vacations…start
a family...share with family and friends....maybe
buy another cake? No wait, scratch that last one!!!
But I gotta tell you something....listen up!!!! I can
almost guarantee you that even if I had taken that
bet for a million dollars ten years ago, and knowing
what's was at stake for me to win – I still wouldn't
have put in the time to work hard, eat healthy, and
trade in that fat suit I used to wear.   Not even for
a million bucks! That kind of cash STILL wouldn't
have motivated me, not at all! Maybe I'm strange
or just talking out of my- you- know–what, but I
just know that, back then, I would have probably
agreed to the bet, but I would still try to play the
same game-the game of hiding and binging that
food.   In other words, I'd start all over again,
hiding food here and there, and basically I would
be at square one all over again! My choice would
be to return to the "barely eating 500 calories a day
plan", working out two hours a day and basically

depriving myself for that money! Only to be surrounded by fatty foods later on that night and dig in because I hadn't tamed that hunger beast after all! Or in another scenario, I would lose the weight to get the reward and then gain that mountain of flesh all back… because my heart wasn't in it… my head wasn't screwed on straight. My insides weren't really fixed... only my wallet. You know, like those lotto winners who go on to gamble, spend, and party away all their fortune, I'd be a loser after all-with just a ton of flab left in the bank account!! I'm posting this because I've seen it happen. When you are ready to get healthy and fit, and I mean: TRULY READY- when you are sick and tired of carrying that fat suitcase and heavy suit around… your attitude can change. Even when you think you're ready… you aren't. Because let me tell you just how much you have to go through to finally... JUST FINALLY… reach the point that NO matter what it takes, you're gonna commit to doing it!!! I'm not saying that sometimes the winners on those weight loss reality TV shows don't succeed in keeping weight off for good. In fact, whenever the old "winners" come back to for appearances on various TV shows, have you noticed that they never look the same as when they hit the BIG WIN before? They always seem to come back a little heavier. I'm not saying it isn't hard... no! Because keeping it off is truly the hard part. But what I'm saying is, to ask people to lose that much just for a prize and a competition... That's just the outside appearance! Have they really worked on themselves INSIDE as well as on the outside? What keeps them from grabbing the junk food again the next time they're alone and the TV audience is gone? My whole point to this confessional tonight is this: if you are at the lowest of the lows... the rock bottom of the rock bottoms...start from there!! Get up and just DO IT for you. Be ready for you and nothing else. Let YOURSELF be that freaking prize!!

*   *   *

Fat Confessional #47:

(can't fit in)

Ain't this the total truth?? When I first met my fellow workout buddies I realized that I hadn't really thought about the fact that, yes, I was touching lives and helping others, and that felt really good! But I started to realize just how much my life was being improved as well. Somehow, I've never felt as if I belonged anywhere! I was always identified as the fat blob of an older sister of two younger beauties. That's reality for the fat chick! And I always felt like an imposter in the world...like a Marilyn Manson floating in a sea of Britney Spears girls! You can't work on the outside without simultaneously working on the inside as well. I never knew that concept! How can I reach out to others, to make a place for myself in the group, if I can't help myself?? That was my mission this year-2013. And as the holiday season and 2014 approaches, I am sitting here in absolute amazement at everything I have accomplished this year and everything that is to come! Thank you to my most amazing Team for helping me to believe in myself enough to kick the weight off my body and for helping me get that confidence I so desperately needed so I can encourage others to start their journey!

*   *   *

Fat Confessional #48:

(save your fat clothes Cait)

Jeans that I won't hide... big baggy jeans that I'll never donate or throw away. Jeans that tell the story, chapter and verse! I'll keep them for the rest of my life to remind me that I'm a fighter in the big battle... the story that I lost half my body weight the healthy way! Reminding me how I felt when I decided "enough was enough" and my excuses and "poor me" had finally run out. These jeans remind me that the odds were stacked against me. And that I took those odds and made those odds my bitch.

*   *   *

Fat Confessional #49:

(fries with that)

Some of you have read or heard this from me before, but I wanted to repost it for those of you who haven't!   Because maybe you've done this before and I just want you to know you're not alone. Here goes! " WOULD YOU LIKE FRIES WITH THAT???" With what??? Yeah, I basically had that conversation in the fast food drive thru every night during those" fat suit days" because, let's face it. My life was a life in the FAST FOOD

77

LANE, and fast food was my food pyramid. We all heard the story of how I would stuff the burgers into my pants when I worked at the restaurant, and don't forget how I would sneak into the bathroom at the tender age of 15 and slam EVERY ONE of those burgers down my throat as if I was about to leave for a "Survivor" shoot! But I have to confess that what I'm least proud of is this: after I stopped working there my love for their fast food menu items NEVER ended. As a teenager, I would find myself sitting in the car, my palms sweaty with anticipation over what I would order that night! Night after night! "Bad things come in three's"! I'm sure you've heard that saying before. Well, this was no different. I was never satisfied with just one bag of my burger meal... I had to order at least THREE MEALS to satisfy my cravings. And I fooled myself (and them, I thought), because, even though I preferred the double burger with cheese and the diet coke, I included two other drinks in the order! Not because I was crazy thirsty for three drinks, but because I wanted to trick them into thinking the three meals were for THREE DIFFERENT PEOPLE, NOT JUST FOR ME!! Yeah, I actually cared what people thought about me and I was disgusted with myself. So it was all an act to help me cope. The acting got better and better, too! I would really get into the role-always smiling at the person in drive thru, asking for a drink holder and extra napkins/ketchup-- you name it. And I almost always made a point of saying something like, "Can I get extra napkins because the kids get so messy?" An Oscar-winning performance! Too bad there was no audience to appreciate my acting skills! Too bad I was referring to me and only me. I would consume all –there were no kids to share the meals with-just me! But I wasn't done yet! There would be the addition of the apple pies and maybe an ice cream shake or two –the perfect ending to my feast! And keep in mind: despite the gorging, within 2 hours I would be hungry again!! I would toss the extra drinks in the trashcan because there was nobody to consume them- I only cared about the diet drink, remember? Amazing the lengths I went to then! Just for that addiction! It's insane!! But I know I'm not alone in this. So thanks for letting me get it off my chest-again!!!

* * *

Fat Confessional #49:

(Dearly Beloved)

Dearly beloved, we are all gathered here today to say "GOODBYE!" to something we once held so close to us. Not that we want to do so, but we just didn't know how to get rid of it once and for all. I'm referring to my old "Fat Suit", of course. I held that fat as close to me as you would hold your child, but yet I didn't hold onto it out of love! No, I held on tight because of something else! FEAR! That's the real reason-fear-the fear you've read about in my previous posts! It was FEAR OF THE UNKNOWN, my unknown future! That's a big part of it! After all, a chick who had never been healthy and healed inside and out, beautiful and strong inside and out, that chick had NO IDEA what steps to take to get there! The only steps I really knew how to take were those going to my fridge to see what I could stuff myself with!! So, "Dearly beloved ", we are also gathered here today to say goodbye to being UNCOMFORTABLE! Do you know one of the things my mom always tells me is how I always looked so uncomfortable, constantly tugging at my clothes and pulling my shirt down as far over my waist as possible! I remember how I always placed a couch pillow in my lap while watching TV, just to conceal the fat underneath, as if a small couch pillow could hide it all-push it away for awhile at least! Yes, I was constantly tugging at my clothes, my bra straps, my pants as if I had an enormous full body "wedgie"! Inside or out, I was never contented and comforted! Always this beautiful, boisterous soul trapped inside a very obese girl who was so unsure of herself and the decisions she was making in life. I still to this very day sometimes tug my shirt down and double-check my bra to make sure there isn't flab hanging over the straps! Even though I know it's gone, I'm still shocked that it is. Crazy! And this journey has taken me SUCH a long time, that I'm still adjusting and taking it all in-especially the accomplishments I've made!! And yet the fat girl in me is still always there in the back of my head! She's still a part of me and honestly, I love her to death! I really love her! No matter how poor her self esteem and confidence level was! I love her spirit, her tenacity, and I love her "Enough with the fat suit" decision! So for you who are still waiting for "ENOUGH!", maybe just make your decision to say "enough!" to be alive longer, do it to be able to throw out those bottles of medicine, or to teach your kids the healthy way to live. Just don't wait too long because you honestly have no idea what life is without that suit on! And I can tell you first hand...Life without your "fat suit" is going to be amazing!

Fat Confessional #50:

(old me)

Just finishing a workout in my living room! And I can't help thinking back to my very first workout... man- oh- man, was it bad!! Think "day 1" of the Biggest Loser workouts...dry heaving, sweat all over the floor, practically, and more dry panting than a dog park run! And it's sad to say that it was only 8 minutes of actually "working out" that I had done! 8 minutes!   And did I mention it was JUST walking!? That's right, my friends, it was 8 minutes of the WORST TORTURE EVER!! The WORST! I remember after that workout, I went through half of box of tissues and cried my eyes out, not because I was so happy that I actually moved off the couch... but I cried because I had let myself get that way. My getting morbidly obese was only my doing! My choice! The stretch marks, the cellulite, the scarily pounding nonstop heart in my chest, the chafed thighs and knee pain was all because I loved to eat and had no idea how to control myself! Did I dare do another workout? Could I?   In the privacy of my living room of course, (there was NO freakin' way I was hitting the gym yet), and I didn't for a long time!! In fact, could I have walked outside? Yup… did I try it? Yup… but I stopped the day some pimple- faced jerks drove past me, mooing like a cow, laughing as they quickly rolled up their windows and peeled away! My living room would do just fine, thank you very much!! Yeah, I might not have completed the entire 20 minute workout DVD that I eagerly placed in my DVD player, but 8 minutes is all it took for me to realize just how important it was for me to do complete that 20 minutes: day in and day out, until I could do more. I was never and I mean NEVER, EVER the active type! I never played sports and I loved the comfort of my pink bedroom so much that it seemed like I hardly ever left it! I hid there with my cassette player, with the New Kids singing on their Block, with the Debbie Gibson beat! My world was in my bedroom! No one could get me out of there for long! So, that workout was a huge shock to this former fat chick's system. It was the start of my journey out of the old pink bedroom!! … So my point in this confessional is… it doesn't matter what exercise or DVD you do! Everybody has a starting point. It's not easy to start! Just look at me, at my story! In fact, it's the hardest thing ever. But if you don't start somewhere you won't ever truly know what you CAN become! You wouldn't know that you would be writing daily to wonderful people to help keep them motivated and strong, you wouldn't know that you would be in a magazine and writing a book and that so many would count on you. You wouldn't know just how much YOU matter!! I'm just a normal person who decided that my life and my body was worth the sweat and tears that it takes to lose that much weight. What will it take for you to see that in yourself? If you'd rather just sit on the cough and complain, then be my guest... but while you're sitting there...can you pass me my running shoes? Get started with me now or regret it later!!

*   *   *

Fat Confessional #52:

(4 years)

This is a long one, so keep reading... and I'm sorry for rambling!! I'd like to think I'm very honest with all of you, but the truth is, I'm not. Partially because it's hard to talk about my fat life! And I'm very hard on myself and I'm my own worst critic but... being that this is a confessional and all... I had to share it with you who are the most loyal followers ever! As you may have read in my "Shape" magazine article, or you may have learned my story through questions you've

emailed me, my weight loss journey has taken me four long LONG years. It's always hard for me to admit that and not just because of the number 4 in four long years… but because of what that number represents for me. Back on that fateful day when I had decided enough was enough, I truly had no idea where to begin. Getting started appeared so scary and overwhelming to me that I was frighteningly clueless… especially with
WHAT to feed myself… which is why my diet was so drastic at first! I thought that being drastic was the only way to get the job done! Getting that dreaded fat that clung to my body as if they were "bffs" getting it OFF!! Where to start?? I didn't research anything, nor did I ask for any advice. At first, I decided to cut my calories immediately-not just by a little, but by a whole lot! Not even thinking twice about it or the effects of that on my body when all I could think of was "skinny -skinny -skinny"!! I cut my calorie intake from trillions to 600. 600 CALORIES A DAY! Can you believe it?? Looking back, I wonder how the heck I did it. I was determined and desperate for a change, period, and that was all that counted! Not the calories, but that!! So, to get started, I only ate things that were pre- portioned because, who had time to learn how to cook healthy and plan a good menu anyways! Combine eating 600 calories a day to 900 calories on "cheat days", followed by 2-3 hours of

only cardio and what do you get?? I'll tell you what you get: a severely starved girl who dropped 180 pounds in a year and a half...insane, right?! Not the way to go about it!! When that year and a half was over, my clothes hung loosely and I was down to almost 129 pounds! My muscle tone was no muscle tone at all! I had no idea what weights were unless I was referring to the weight carried on my 5'4 frame!! I remember the day I weighed myself and saw that big glowing 129 looking at me! What do you think was my first thought?? I thought with excitement: "I'M CURED!" I literally said, "HOLY CRAP, I'M CURED...IVE CURED MYSELF!! Because I thought I had fought the battle and won it and that I could go back to doing whatever I wanted, including eating whatever, WHATEVER I wanted!! And it would never, ever creep back on me. Boy was I WRONG!!!!! I completely stopped working out, like I mean COMPLETELY! I went out every night with friends and started gorging on the same crummy fast food stuff as if it was going out of style! And in a matter of 4 months, I had gained 70 pounds back. OH NO, 70 POUNDS-back on my body again!! Was I miserable and depressed because months later I had gained back all that I had lost? Yes, because I WASN'T CURED AFTER ALL! By now I had thrown all of my fat clothes out... I had done my skinny dance and showed myself off to the world and now I had to go

BACK into hiding. So basically-I DID! I became a hermit again! I went nowhere…canceled all my party plans with friends and skipped the RSVPs because I was so humiliated that I had done this to myself-AGAIN!! I truly thought that just crash dieting could solve my problems. But I didn't realize that an entire LIFESTYLE CHANGE along with a healthy thought process was needed to change my life. For good!! Thank God I've realized that now… but it's taken me 2 more years now to get to that full realization. It's taken me all of 32 years to finally love myself, no matter where I jiggle and no matter how much I shake. I hope this touches you somewhere out there and that you realize that you do not need to be so drastic to get results. You just need to believe it can be done! And to love yourself and realize that you are worth the lifestyle change. Good exercise, (in my case, beginning a weight and resistance routine), and eating healthy really does get you the results that will last forever… deprivation does not!

*   *   *

Fat Confessional #53:

(when Monday comes)

To the quitters… to the starters and the stoppers… to the "when Monday comes I'll do it" group… I feel it is in my best interest to give you these words. I feel the strongest connection with you because I was (pick the best answer!): A. a QUITTER, B. a starter and stopper, C. a "When Monday comes my healthy diet starts" excuser, D. All of the above. The answer? I was D!!!! I always "went hard" or at least I thought I had been a go- getter, but then again, I never noticed any sweat coming out of my pores! But anyway, I would go hard and heavy, and then quit a few days later. Throw the largest pity party out there that would make any Debbie Downer jealous! Then I would "Wait for Monday" and start all over again. Why we pick Mondays is beyond my rational thinking! Poor Monday gets all the bad press! But I'm speaking to you because you need to hear it just the same! There is nobody out there who can get that fat off your body other than you. NOBODY!!! Quit whining and throwing tantrums about how much you want to change and then continue to NOT to do anything about it. I know these words are harsh, but man- oh- man, if only someone had uttered these words to me (well, they probably did, but I wasn't in that zone!) So the truth hurts but... IT'S STILL THE TRUTH! So quit! Just stop it! Quit lying to yourself when you say you're ready, because chances are, you aren't! How do I know that? Because if you were ready to get started, you'd already be doing something about it. It's not easy... you know that by now. But CHAMPIONS AREN'T MADE ON THE COUCH, PEOPLE! The bottom line is this: you will finally run out of excuses... and Mondays... and special occasions... and "I'll do it tomorrow!"... and you'll face the truth that this has to be 100% for the REST OF YOUR LIFE!! If you're STILL perfectly content being envious of others lives while you click away at the remote and curse when the batteries run out... well then, by all means, have it. But you know it's in you to change your focus... just like I knew it was in me! So pick the gym floor or the hospital floor, people... and quit "not doing" something about it!!! Don't you want to be proud of yourself and feel beautiful not just inside but also out? Don't you want to live a long life with your family? Because if MAC 'N CHEESE is worth more than what you have to offer yourself and others, then be my guest and go for it!! But while you're complaining... and hating yourself... I'll be tackling obstacles and changing lives, and not just my own. You can do this, people!!! This is not impossible! It's in your hands!!

*   *   *

Fat Confessional #54:

(weddings)

Don't you just love weddings? I never lose that
fascination for those white dresses and flowers! Well,
we have a friend's wedding event next weekend and I
needed to buy a dress for it... so today that is what I
set out to do. Driving to the mall with all my old "fat
girl rules" in my head: You remember those rules:
NO WHITE CLOTHES... white fabric makes you
look big-BIG! Like a HUGE marshmallow, or better
yet, the "Michelin Man" (I've actually been called that
before!) So better stay away from white! Then there's
the "No patterns, stripes, or large prints" rule.
"Caitlin, just stay away from patterns," I repeated to
myself. "They make you look too noticeable in a
crowd."   I would continue with the rest of the rules:
"Please, no horizontal stripes, either... then you look
wider than you actually are. And if you have to do
stripes, just go with diagonals- you'll be ok with those!
And nothing that clings to your body, please! Instead,
find the baggiest looking dress possible so that way it
hides your shape!! " Bla-bla-bla! Replaying these

rules on a daily basis used to be the way I chose to live. I say chose because I chose to eat a large pizza by myself and I chose not to work out. Which means I then chose to "write" those rules for myself. I gotta tell you that it's such a relief to throw those rules away, to have 20 dresses to choose from in a fitting room and have a hard time deciding because they ALL look good on you! Never again do I need to follow those old commands, which leaves me more time to focus on the more important things... like sitting back and smelling the roses now that the cake batter smell has faded away!! I need to take the time to really appreciate myself and all the hard work I've done. I keep thinking it hasn't really happened-is it really true that I've come this far in achieving my goals?? Yes, it is true! I get those little reminders, like the one today when the sales girl at a dress boutique asked me if I wanted to go to the other side of the store. Apparently, I wandered into the "plus size section" and forgot that I didn't need to be there-not anymore, for obvious reasons. It's still a habit that I hit those areas first because for almost 30 years of my life I had to!! Man, does it feel good to take those old rules and shove them. NO MORE RULES and OBSTACLES!!! P.S. I found my dress and it looks fantastic!!

* * *

Fat Confessional #55:

(holidays)

T'was the night before Christmas, when all through
the house,
my thoughts were on stuffing candy down my already
tight blouse…

  our stockings were hung on our mantle with care,
in the hopes that Santa, and not Cait, would be there.
My siblings all nestled, tucked in their warm beds,
while I lay awake with chocolate stuck in my head.
Suddenly, in her room, there arose such a clatter,
as Cait sprang out of her bed, hungry for cake batter!
She was dressed in tight sweatpants- fat suit starting to
show -

  as Cait crept quietly downstairs like a pro.
Her eyes how they sparkled, while she eyed her prize,
those lovely stuffed stockings, hung way up high.
Her mission was clear on that fateful night…
"I need to get those stockings and not cause a fright!"
As she tip- toed upstairs, she was proud of her find,
for now there was chocolate to ease her hungry mind!!
Cait dumped out the stockings on her pink cotton
sheets...

and stared at the wrappers so shiny, so many treats!
Cait carefully selected each morsel she saw,

then realized she needed to leave some... maybe leave them all!

For her siblings "would never do this to you, Cait," she thought.

They would never sneak into her stocking that night! But Merry Christmas to all and to all a good BITE!!

Yes, I am totally guilty of this!! To my younger siblings, I'm saying I'm sorry, and to my parents as well! Sorry for always sneaking downstairs in the middle of the night- every Christmas eve! For all of these things I apologize: A. Eating all the cookies for "Santa" B. drinking all his milk C. taking all the "best" candy from your stockings before you even knew about it or D. all of the above.. MY ANSWER IS D!!!!!!! I AM GUILTY OF BEING A STOCKING THIEF!!! Just call me "stocking stuffer" because I would sneak downstairs and stuff myself with what was in our stockings!! Thank God that's over! Thank God that's off my chest-in both meanings!!!

* * *

Fat Confessional #56

(school days)

Wearing that dress today to the wedding (remember my previous post about the wedding dress?) well, that made me feel amazing… why?? Because I haven't had a dress on in years before I downsized myself! I was never one to wear dresses before and not even skirts… not after what happened on that fateful day. You will want to know what I'm talking about, I suppose. So let me dust off the old memory box and share this story with you. It was dark there, well, there were some flashing lights and smoke machines in the place, but other than that it was dark. "Ace of Base" was blaring on the sound system. It was 1994, after all, and "Don't Turn Around" was a big deal!!!! Yep, it was 1994 and I was at a school dance, believe it or not! Dare I go and even dream I'd be asked to dance?? Heck no. I went because I wanted to get out of my house and hang out with the handful of friends I had. My mom thought it would be appropriate that I wear a skirt since it was a dance, so we found an outfit. And I went, but not with a smile on my face, I have to add! I hated skirts because they showed off my thunder thighs, of course!! But that wasn't all… I also wore a 1990's shirt with long sleeves and a matching vest! Remember when vests were cool?!?!?!?! Or maybe they never were, but whatever!

Well, I was sitting in a chair, desperately wanting to dance, when "Heavy D" came on and this girl, meaning me, decided to break into dance and I mean hardcore dance, complete with arms flying around and all that! I was trying to do the "running man dance" but what ended up happening was that my skirt split- yes, SPLIT- completely down the back all the way to my rear!! I didn't realize it til I felt a major draft of cold air back there, and had to run out quickly before my "granny panties" were on display for the entire school to see. Another 6th grade experience like the "faceplant in the mud" I had when I fell on the volleyball field during gym class that year. Good times my friends... good times!

* * *

Fat Confessional #57:

(had a bad day)

We've all had those days! You know, those days when you wake up feeling bloated, feeling fat and suddenly nothing fits or looks good! Your hair looks lank and limp no matter how much you style it, even your makeup and skin looks bad! What do we call those days?? I think the phrase is "Fat days", when you feel just ugly! Maybe "feeling like crap days" works better! Well, have you ever had the opposite kind of day?? Ever had a day when you wake up and just feel amazing? Even when sweat is running down the sides of your arms and your breath stinks because who brushes their teeth before the gym anyways... and yet you still feel, well, beautiful??? Even if those jeans don't fit right and you have "flyaway hair"... and yet, you still think you're gorgeous anyway??? Today is that kind of day for me! I'm having a pretty day and I want to shout it from the roof tops! I don't think I've ever had a really pretty day in my life to be honest with you... I've had great hair days or gorgeous skin days but I've never just been perfectly content no matter what my appearance was. But today THAT day is mine! I've earned it too! I've earned this damn pretty day and I'm gonna make sure I rock the hell out of it. It's taken me 32 years of hard living to get this day, so it had better last! I eat healthy not because I'm crazy... but because now I know how to eat to feel better! And not only that, to look better and to live longer also! I know how my body feels when I eat badly (just ask me how Christmas day was) and I have finally figured out my nutrition wants and needs-how to make them the SAME THING!! I work out because I love my life and want to live a long one and if you don't love yourself enough to want to feel this way I feel so sorry for you... you're truly missing out! Coming from the girl who needed a butt- load of makeup on her double chins, and baggy clothes to cover her fat rolls... to now feeling pretty in sweat pants with sweaty hair sticking to her face..I'd say that's a WIN situation! So go on... do something good for yourself and feel pretty!

$$* \quad * \quad *$$

Fat Confessional #58:

(choose your fit)

How do you choose your fitness? Think about it! Remember gazing at all the fitness workout DVDs in the sporting goods sections at the local retail stores and thinking... "Ok what will be easy enough for me to do, yet will hold my attention so I don't quit and give up? An "Easy" rating for a workout DVD for a 332 pound female who grew up hating sports and loving french fries meant "EXTREMELY, EXTREMELY EASY". But for some reason I would shell out ridiculous amounts of money on programs and then never use them. Never! I distinctly remember sitting on my couch, pillow in lap to hide the belly, with the remote in my hand and a can of sour cream and onion chips perched on my lap... ALL THE WHILE WATCHING A FITNESS

PROGRAM to see if it was "easy" enough for me to do! Did I really do that?? YES I DID!!! It's hilarious if you picture it, but really that was my day–to- day life. "Easy way out Cait" was my real identity! Easy way out for everything! "But that's too much work for me," I'd say to myself. "I know I can lose the weight but that takes up too much time, work and effort to do that! I would have preferred some Channing Tatum look-alike Prince Charming to come along and use his magic wand to hide my fat suit. Let someone else do it! That's what my thoughts were. I spent countless days stalking the sporting goods sections at my favorite retail stores, always trying to fill that void and find the answer to what I was missing in my life! I even remember the check out girl giggling and looking at me funny when I bought some of these workouts. Did she have trouble thinking I'd be actually using these workouts? Because she knew, as well as I knew, that the real deal was that those plastic-wrapped DVDs would sit on my shelf and gather dust instead. BUT, OH WAIT...That's right… I FINALLY DID IT!! I peeled that wrapper off a DVD one day and decided to: A. stop being a (excuse my french) bullshitter B. get with the program and get off the couch C. quit lying and pointing fingers at everyone else in the world for my issues, and D. take matters into my own hands and work this fat off my body. So I started with the easiest workout I could find-but considering that a leisure walk down the street made me practically dry heave my lunch... that was really all I could do at the time. Fast forward to NOW: How do I stay motivated at this point?? Take it day by day! You just do! It's your life! You wake up every day and you live. You live each day better than the day before. That's it! Why waste your time on this earth with food stuffed in your mouth and feeling that awful envy of the lives of all those lucky girls you see out in the world? Why not YOU? You be the one people are jealous about! Why can't you be the one that gets those admiring looks from the guys? Why not? You can be the one who's able to run after your 3- year - old without practically passing out on the floor. The one who has it all together in a nice life!! Aren't you worth it?? I know I was worth that! It took me long enough to realize it... BUT I KNOW THAT I WAS WORTH THE TIME IT TOOK!

*   *   *

Fat Confessional #59:

(the old me gets a message)

What would I say to my 22 year- old- self if I could
speak to her? Would I say this: that life is better than
it is for you at this moment, that one day you'll be
strong, one day you won't cry over the scale? I would
repeat again and again, that one day you won't cry at
the mirror or watch others with miserable envy eating
you inside! That someday soon it's a great day
because you'll start a new path and never stop! That's
the day you'll say, "I feel beautiful in and beautiful
out," and you'll truly mean it! That's the time you'll
reach for the stars...put them in your pocket and
never let them go!

* * *

Fat Confessional #60

(12 step for fat Cait)

For some of you this is familiar, but for not for others.
And for some of you this IS you but you're in denial
and don't want to admit it! So for now, just think of
this confessional as the "twelve step program for
emotional eaters" OK? Because I was one, and some

of you are too. Here goes: If you have ever lied or cheated for food, raise your hand!! Check yes! I'm sure you have, time and time again. Oh but, I barely ate today… that's a good one-something I've said so many freakin' times!   I barely ate lunch or breakfast so I'm going to have this huge heaping bowl of pasta for dinner, because I deserve it. Clearly knowing in the back of your head exactly what you ate all day and that you certainly aren't starving. You just wanted the heaping bowl of pasta IN ADDITION TO all the rest of the meals! Ok, let's continue: Have you ever felt guilty about the food you've eaten??   Raise your hand if you have. I admit it- I have! Many, many times! In fact, it's hard for me to type this confessional with one hand raised, but it's the truth. Next: Note to self if you have to stuff food in your pockets to sneak it somewhere and eat it! Well, that's not a good thing either! Own up, Cait! OK I will: What kinds of foods have been stuffed in my pockets??? Pretty much anything but soup!! Never did figure that one out! But my favorite pocket foods were, guess what?? CUPCAKES, COOKIES AND anything from the bakery section of a grocery store, but getting the "icing evidence" away was tricky! That one took a little planning, maybe like grabbing three or four napkins and wrapping them around my treasures! Fast Food burgers, well, that was an easier pocket food back then. Remember my earlier post about starting at age 15 working for a fast food place? I posted about how I got good at stuffing the burgers and breakfast treats in my pants so I could eat them later after work? And have you ever gone to the sandwich or sub shop and stuffed an extra 6 inch beauty in your pocket? I have! Really?? YEP I HAVE!!! Don't forget the cookies you get for dessert too! They're easy to hide in any pocket or even the wasteband of your jeans or pants! My now- famous "fat jeans" that still hang in my closet to this day remind me daily of that! (don't worry, they ARE clean!) The bottom line is: that food you've been hiding is good for 2.5 seconds! That's all! After that, you're already onto your next craving! Though I'm not a scientist and I can't possibly tell you what goes through your mind during a binge, but it's truly insane how you get under the spell of that "hiding food" life! It's like murder without all the blood. There is no stopping you when you're in that mindframe. You will do what it takes…ANYTHING! Think lions with saliva dripping from sharp teeth… yep, that was me on a binge. My addiction ruled me and I was in a constant state of binging! As I posted yesterday about the store cashier who asked me: "How did you get so big?? Easy!! The answer is easy: "FOOD. FOOD. FOOD!!" No, I wasn't BIG BONED like I led others to believe as if a skeleton could be fat. JUST SO MUCH DENIAL when you are an

emotional eater. You may even think, "I'm over it!"
But then here comes your" trigger food" walking all
sass and swagger right up to you and in your face!
And before you know it, you're back again in BINGE-
LAND! You're KNEE DEEP in stuffed crust pizza
from that pizza restaurant! Yes, raise your hand if you
have eaten a whole pie to yourself (raises hand), and
raise your hand if you're ready to tackle this problem
once and for all.....is it RAISED???? Ok, now go
ahead, move out of BINGE-LAND and fix it! You
are the problem-- but you are also the solution! Keep
that in mind every day!!

*   *   *

Fat Confessional #61:

(hate selfies)

Yes, it's hard to post photos of myself from the "FAT
DAYS," but I pride myself in being honest with you
all. That's important to me! So when I post pics of
me in my granny panties, I'm doing that to show you
that they are falling off me now! And that is
awesome! Is my body perfect?? Nope. I still have

stretch marks. I still have cellulite. I still have loose skin. But the difference is that I don't care! This body got me to the point I'm at today. It's these legs that have taken the steps from that farthest parking spot- instead of the closer one in the store lot. It's these legs that have walked and run a million miles... these legs that took the stairs up four floors instead of the easy elevator. It's this body that chose to do it the hard way and never once gave up. I love this body- we've been through a lot together! And I have all those battle wounds left to remind me that I don't ever want to fight that battle again. Never!

Not only have I lost this weight, but I've lost the insecurities...I have lost the pain...I have lost the uncomfortable feelings of self loathing and always wanting to be someone else!   What a feeling! It goes on and on! So the next time you're tired and saying "poor me:" The next time you are out of breath... and want to give up... remember how good it can feel if you just keep on going!

* * *

Fat Confessional #62:

(BREAD BREAD BREAD)

I know it's not Wednesday, the day I've always posted my "Fat Confessionals"… but I had to get this out now before I forget about it and don't think to share it with you! So tonight after work, my friend and I ran to the grocery store to pick up some more eggs… we go through lots in my household. We walked past the bread section to get to the back of the store where the eggs are located. Going past I saw one of my former FAVES!! There it is: The POTATO BREAD! If you aren't a fan, you more than likely won't enjoy this story. But I was a huge fan and still am to this day. I remembered way back when…I would buy WHOLE LOAVES OF THAT delicious bread- FOR MYSELF!! And I would butter piece after piece and lay them all out on a plate with a tall glass of milk. I would take in the sight, then CHOW DOWN! That was THE snack, my huge treat!! I also remember taking one piece of bread and rolling it into a ball and eating many, many little balls of bread that way as well! Looking at today, I feel relieved that things have changed so much! I cannot even think about doing that now… can't even believe I did those things. I can't believe that JUST 30 minutes later after eating many slices of that bread, sometimes a WHOLE LOAF… I would be hungry all over again. For those of you who struggle with binge eating or emotional eating, there is hope! Hope for a future that's free of binging and stuffing! Trust in yourself, be strong, and have lots of faith that good changes will happen... and one day it just might! Needless to say I didn't buy any of the potato bread tonight! And the english muffins almost tempted me to grab a few of those with cinnamon raisins... I still struggle and work at it! But I stayed strong, Hurray!!

*   *   *

Fat Confessional #63

(FACTS)

These were a few of my favorite things... FACT: I would sit on my couch with an entire tube of chocolate chip cookie dough... after cutting the end from the wrapper with scissors, I would sit with a spoon and eat the entire thing... in ONE sitting! FACT: I would buy container after container of icing for cakes and I would sit on my couch and spoon-feed myself the entire container. My stomach would ache and cramp afterwards and I always felt so horribly guilty for doing it. But the taste of that stuff would drive me crazy. I literally think about doing that every

106

time I see those colorful little containers in the grocery store to this day!! And I literally know that if I were to binge on those icings again, I would continue making other bad choices and take a rolling tumble down that steep hill. And why is it that we are drawn to making those poor choices? Why is it that with one very bad choice, many more come right after it?? We do it… we give up… we throw in the towel and jump in the guilt. Then the next day we work out hard, get sweaty, and pretend it didn't happen! What Icing? I didn't eat that junk! Why do we sabotage ourselves in such a way? I'm not a scientist and I only wish I knew the answers to the questions I have and that so many of you have as well. I'm just grateful I know how to push those old emo feelings about foods away now. It's not easy at all but it's something that has to be done and done on a daily basis. EVERY DAY! We are only human after all, and we're prone to taking bad turns in the road! Taking our eyes off the wheel, we drive and slip into the ditch! So people, change your way of thinking about food… that's the bottom line!! This is not your last meal… and this is not your last supper!! You are not shipping off to "survivor". It's not your last meal! So why eat like that? Look at food differently-EAT TO LIVE, DON'T LIVE TO EAT!!!! Look at food differently--and train your mind to do the same!!

*   *   *

Fat Confessional #64:

(Boobs)

Ok, time for a little "girl talk!" Ok, what's that? Let me talk to you a little bit about my ta ta's... not trying to gross you out or anything, but let's be real here! After going from a 48 E cup... to a 34 C cup... well, they didn't look too pretty. You would think so right? But nope. They basically resembled flat pancakes that were trying to reach my bellybutton and were almost, almost there! I could squeeze them and let go and they would remain the shape of my hand and that's no lie. Without going into the rest of the details, let's just say I was humiliated about the shape of "the girls"! So, bring on the lights and the orchestra!! What was the solution to the flat pancake problem?? What was it??? Two big little words! "BENCH PRESS"!! WOOT WOOT!!!! I gotta tell you that in the almost 5 months since I've started HEAVIER LIFTING AND LESS CARDIO... my boobs have drastically changed!! I may be almost 33 but trust me, my girls look like they are 23. Honest! I never in my life have had nice ta ta's! They were always strapped down with

3 sports bras when working out and I had to pray to the run gods that I wouldn't have a black eye when I first started running. They swept the floor with my bra off and that back pain… the back pain I suffered from carrying around those big girls! But now it's a whole new world. They are perky and I can fit into anything now and I owe it all to chest exercises!! So… thanks for letting me be so "detailed" and never underestimate the power of Iron. For beginners, try the light dumbbells and progress up to heavier weights from there… and trust me, it works!!!

* * *

Fat Confessional #65:

(365 days)

Have you ever sat and thought about just where you were last year? I remember where I was…I do!! I was struggling hard core, stuck on a major plateau that almost wrecked me and this journey of mine. I was sitting in my house feeling totally miserable because my scale was stuck at 193 pounds for months… months and months! What was I not doing, or doing wrong? Then I thought, "Maybe if I just clean up my eating… since I was already doing 5-6 workouts a week! Ya think???? It was obvious that it couldn't be my fitness program that needed work. Yep, maybe that was it! I needed to move to the next step here! So I made the decision to clean up my eating. That was worth a try! And then I decided to create this page. "For me, not for an audience", I thought! I created this page not thinking anybody would pay attention to it, other than a few supportive friends. I'd start this page to help myself by keeping an online diary, and to hold myself accountable. Because if you are an emotional eater and struggling…the act of writing helps tremendously! Well, at least it's helped me and still does to this day. I cannot begin to tell you how much it motivates me when I write these heartfelt words daily. When I see all the struggles and challenges! For today then, look in your past and be thankful for how far you've come in a year! Amazing, isn't it? Celebrate little victories. The fact that you have even started is cause for celebration. Only the strong survive and the weak fail and will fail again. Not many people can do this and really be diligent with their nutrition and fitness. But we all have to start somewhere! So, where were you last year? And what is the best health advice you've ever been given? Would you say you are struggling? Or are you celebrating?

*   *   *

Fat Confessional#66

(no eye contact)

Eyes down to the ground..can't make eye contact with anyone for fear that they will see the pain behind these green eyes of mine. Pain caused by myself and myself only..the pain that was only released with a bag of chips..an entire carton of ben and jerry's..or a cake ordered from the bakery. The pain of never feeling good enough or ever fitting in..funny and laughing on the outside but miserable on the inside. Day in and day out I lived like this..I was absolutely knocking on deaths door..and in fact even sometimes eager to check and see if it was open. Always feeling alone and never thinking my life would ever change. Always depending on others to fix it for me and when they couldn't I would cut ties and turn to food again.

Today walking into the grocery store I caught a guy looking at me and thought oh god is there something on my face? Or maybe toilet paper stuck to my flip flops? What the heck is he even looking at me for..there's way better looking people inside this store so umm what the what? It hit me that maybe I was worthy of these stolen glances? Maybe my hard work has paid off and I am actually attractive to the public?

If you've never been morbidly obese as I have well you can't possibly understand my way of thinking..but regardless of what you all see in my photos when I post them..I will never view myself that way...these very photos attached to this post is how I still often view myself. It's so hard to explain..I know my clothes are smaller and that I can see my feet..I know that my thighs don't rub together and that I no longer need to sleep with a pillow in between them. I know that when I'm out to dinner I can sit really close to the table now..I know that my energy is thru the mother effing roof...I know that I'm happy and feel fantastic. But sometimes just sometimes I see this girl. The girl that most certainly did receive a ton of stares growing up...but not for the right reasons. So to the guy in the grocery store that "checked me out"...you are welcome! I worked so damn hard for this you can stare all you want! Even if I won't stare back.

* * * * * *

If you've learned anything from reading this book, you've learned that you are not alone in this! I was in your shoes not so long ago, and I hit my rock bottom! Minus 190 pounds later, I am a different person-a better person, with a new life ahead! For my followers who are struggling, I wish the same for each and every one of you! So, look for my blogs on facebook.com/eatrunliftrepeat and eatrunliftrepeat.com for inspiration and encouragement! Also look for more books in the future. I'm a normal chick that lost a lot of weight but we all struggle day in and day out. What's important is that you start and do not stop!!! You got this?

www.ingramcontent.com/pod-product-compliance
Lightning Source LLC
Chambersburg PA
CBHW050537280326
41933CB00011B/1615